Also Available From the American Academy of Pediatrics

Common Conditions

ADHD: What Every Parent Needs to Know

Allergies and Asthma: What Every Parent Needs to Know

My Child Is Sick! Expert Advice for Managing Common Illnesses and Injuries

Sleep: What Every Parent Needs to Know

Waking Up Dry: A Guide to Help Children Overcome Bedwetting

Developmental, Behavioral, and Psychosocial Information

Autism Spectrum Disorders: What Every Parent Needs to Know

CyberSafe: Protecting and Empowering Kids in the Digital World of Texting, Gaming, and Social Media

Mental Health, Naturally: The Family Guide to Holistic Care for a Healthy Mind and Body

Newborns, Infants, and Toddlers

Caring for Your Baby and Young Child: Birth to Age 5*

Dad to Dad: Parenting Like a Pro

Guide to Toilet Training*

Heading Home With Your Newborn: From Birth to Reality

Mommy Calls: Dr. Tanya Answers Parents' Top 101 Questions About Babies and Toddlers

New Mother's Guide to Breastfeeding*

Newborn Intensive Care: What Every Parent Needs to Know

Raising Twins: From Pregnancy to Preschool

Retro Baby: Cut Back on All the Gear and Boost Your Baby's Development With More Than 100 Time-tested Activities

Your Baby's First Year*

Nutrition and Fitness

Food Fights: Winning the Nutritional Challenges of Parenthood Armed With Insight, Humor, and a Bottle of Ketchup

Nutrition: What Every Parent Needs to Know

A Parent's Guide to Childhood Obesity: A Road Map to Health

Sports Success R$_x$! Your Child's Prescription for the Best Experience

School-aged Children and Adolescents

Building Resilience in Children and Teens: Giving Kids Roots and Wings

Caring for Your School-Age Child: Ages 5 to 12

Caring for Your Teenager

Less Stress, More Success: A New Approach to Guiding Your Teen Through College Admissions and Beyond

For more information, please visit the official AAP Web site for parents, www.HealthyChildren.org/bookstore.

*This book is also available in Spanish.

Mama Doc Medicine

Finding Calm and Confidence in Parenting,
Child Health, and Work-Life Balance

Wendy Sue Swanson, MD, MBE, FAAP
Pediatrician, Mom, Advocate, Author

American Academy of Pediatrics
DEDICATED TO THE HEALTH OF ALL CHILDREN™

American Academy of Pediatrics Department of Marketing and Publications Staff

Director, Department of Marketing and Publications
Maureen DeRosa, MPA

Manager, Editorial Services
Jason Crase

Director, Division of Product Development
Mark Grimes

Publishing and Production Services Specialist
Shannan Martin

Manager, Consumer Publishing
Carolyn Kolbaba

Manager, Art Direction and Production
Linda Diamond

Manager, Digital Strategy and Product Development
Jeff Mahony

Director, Division of Marketing and Sales
Julia Lee

Coordinator, Product Development
Holly Kaminski

Manager, Consumer Marketing and Sales
Kathleen Juhl

Director, Division of Publishing and Production Services
Sandi King, MS

Manager, Consumer Product Marketing
Mary Jo Reynolds

Published by the American Academy of Pediatrics
141 Northwest Point Blvd, Elk Grove Village, IL 60007-1019
847/434-4000
Fax: 847/434-8000
www.aap.org

Cover design by R. Scott Rattray
Cover photo © Janet Klinger Photography
Dr Swanson head shot by Amos Morgan
Book design by Linda Diamond
Infographics design by Killer Infographics Inc.

Library of Congress Control Number: 2013943971
ISBN: 978-1-58110-837-8
eISBN: 978-1-58110-832-3

The recommendations in this publication do not indicate an exclusive course of treatment or serve as a standard of medical care. Variations, taking into account individual circumstances, may be appropriate.

Statements and opinions expressed are those of the author and not necessarily those of the American Academy of Pediatrics.

Products and Web sites are mentioned for informational purposes only. Inclusion in this publication does not imply endorsement by the American Academy of Pediatrics. The American Academy of Pediatrics is not responsible for the content of the resources mentioned in this publication. Web site addresses are as current as possible but may change at any time.

Every effort is made to keep *Mama Doc Medicine: Finding Calm and Confidence in Parenting, Child Health, and Work-Life Balance* consistent with the most recent advice and information available from the American Academy of Pediatrics.

Portions of the book are from original blog posts written by Dr Wendy Sue Swanson, pediatrician and author of Seattle Mama Doc, a Seattle Children's Hospital blog, copyright Seattle Children's Hospital; used with permission. www.seattlemamadoc.com

CB0075
9-341   1 2 3 4 5 6 7 8 9 10

What People Are Saying

———⚜———

A funny, irreverent, compassionate, and timely guide to how to raise a child in an era when misinformation often rules the day.
— Paul A. Offit, MD, FAAP
 Chief, Division of Infectious Diseases, The Children's Hospital of Philadelphia, and author of *Autism's False Prophets: Bad Science, Risky Medicine, and the Search for a Cure*

———⚜———

I first discovered Wendy Sue Swanson as @SeattleMamaDoc on Twitter. I loved seeing her take on the most important children's health issues of the day. From there I found her terrific blog. Here in one collection is the best of Seattle Mama Doc, evidence-based advice on so many of the questions parents raise. It is packed with practical information; loaded with facts and tips to let you make informed decisions about your child's life. It also contains great advice on balancing your role as a parent with the other things you do in your life. A must-read for new parents!
— Richard Besser, MD, FAAP
 Chief Health and Medical Editor, ABC News, and author of *Tell Me the Truth, Doctor: Easy-to-Understand Answers to Your Most Confusing and Critical Health Questions*

———⚜———

In *Mama Doc Medicine: Finding Calm and Confidence in Parenting, Child Health, and Work-Life Balance,* Dr Swanson effortlessly tackles some of the most difficult and controversial parenting topics with guidance, facts, and real-world examples—leaving you informed and inspired. Life would have been a lot less stressful if my wife and I had had this book when we were starting our family.
— Seth Mnookin
 Associate Director, Graduate Program in Science Writing, Massachusetts Institute of Technology, and author of *The Panic Virus: The True Story Behind the Vaccine-Autism Controversy*

———⚜———

I dare you to read this book and NOT immediately incorporate several new techniques into your parenting style. You'll find yourself continually quoting *Mama Doc Medicine* to family and friends over the course of any given day.

— Michele Borba, EdD

Internationally recognized parenting expert, *Today* show contributor, and author of 22 books, including *The Big Book of Parenting Solutions: 101 Answers to Your Everyday Challenges and Wildest Worries* and *Building Moral Intelligence: The Seven Essential Virtues That Teach Kids to Do the Right Thing*

Dr Swanson has used the tools of the digital age to define herself as one of this generation's most genuine and influential physician voices. *Mama Doc Medicine* delivers actionable, evidence-based information with the type of transparent, reassuring authority that only she can deliver.

— Bryan Vartabedian, MD

Assistant Professor of Pediatrics, Baylor College of Medicine; attending physician, Texas Children's Hospital; and blogger at 33charts.com

I wish I had this book when I was a new mom! Filled with humor and compassion, *Mama Doc Medicine* is a great guide for helping parents navigate all the stages of childhood and not forgetting their own health in the process!

— Laurie David

Author of *The Family Dinner: Great Ways to Connect with Your Kids, One Meal at a Time* and *The Family Cooks: 100+ Recipes Guaranteed to Get Your Family Craving Food That's Simple, Fresh, and Incredibly Good for You* and producer of *Fed Up* and *An Inconvenient Truth*

Offering the perfect mix of experienced pediatrician, empathetic parent, and renowned mom-blogger, new and seasoned parents alike are sure to find this fantastic new book to be as invaluable, insightful, reassuring, and relatable as Dr Wendy Sue herself!

— Laura A. Jana, MD, FAAP

Pediatrician; coauthor of *Heading Home With Your Newborn: From Birth to Reality* and *Food Fights: Winning the Nutritional Challenges of Parenthood Armed With Insight, Humor, and a Bottle of Ketchup;* and founder, Practical Parenting Consulting

Medicine and the digital era are finally converging, and no one could capture that better than Dr Wendy Sue Swanson in *Mama Doc Medicine*. @SeattleMamaDoc is my go-to source on Twitter for pediatric pearls, and this book will undoubtedly be regarded as a treasure trove of best parenting and child health practice. The savvy parent's must-read if there ever was one.

— Eric J. Topol, MD

　　Chief Academic Officer, Scripps Health; Professor of Genomics, The Scripps Research Institute; and author of *The Creative Destruction of Medicine: How the Digital Revolution Will Create Better Health Care*

Dr Wendy Sue Swanson embraces the art and science of children's health and adds a dose of reality for parents who are in the trenches. A must-read for all parents struggling to do their best and maintain their sanity in the process!

— Ari Brown, MD, FAAP

　　Pediatrician and author of *Baby 411: Clear Answers & Smart Advice for Your Baby's First Year*

Pediatrician, mom, and journalist Dr Wendy Sue Swanson put together her greatest tips on everything you ever wanted to know about parenting, ranging from the medical (colic, teething, and ear infections) to the practical (think junk food, TV time, and bouncy houses). For parents, this is the book to grab if you've ever wondered, "What would my pediatrician think about this?" but didn't have time to ask during a short office visit. As a pediatrician, this is the book I wish I had written if I had the time! *Mama Doc Medicine* is full of interesting and sound advice for anyone seeking calm and confidence in parenthood. I highly recommend it!

— Jennifer Shu, MD, FAAP

　　Pediatrician, mom, and coauthor of *Heading Home With Your Newborn: From Birth to Reality* and *Food Fights: Winning the Nutritional Challenges of Parenthood Armed With Insight, Humor, and a Bottle of Ketchup*

—◦◊◦—

Mama Doc Medicine is an insightful and informative collection of Dr Wendy Sue Swanson's wise words on a multitude of topics every parent wants and needs to know to raise a healthy and happy child in today's world of information overload. Her vulnerability as a mom, expertise as a leading pediatrician, status as a social media guru, and candid nature make this book a must-read for any parent, grandparent, or caregiver.
— Tanya Remer Altmann, MD, FAAP
    Pediatrician and author of *Mommy Calls: Dr. Tanya Answers Parents' Top 101 Questions About Babies and Toddlers*

—◦◊◦—

As parents, we all want a partner. We need someone to lean into, a trusted voice to help us make the tough decisions when our minds are too busy spinning, or simply too overwhelmed. Fortunately, Dr Wendy Sue Swanson has arrived. Through personal stories, understandable science, and up-to-date medical evidence, Dr Swanson blends her expertise as a pediatric physician with her experience as a loving parent and wife. Her book offers a well-indexed, reliable, and readable blend of important child health topics, while allowing her true joy in helping families make better decisions for their children leap from every page. Be sure to keep this book close; you will be reaching for the comfort of Dr Swanson's advice over and over again.
— Natasha Burgert, MD, FAAP
    Pediatrician and blogger at kckidsdoc.com

—◦◊◦—

It's hard being a parent—and even harder these days, with all the information overload, not to mention how competitive it can feel. Wendy Sue helps parents sort through all the information and competition, understand what's important, and figure out what's best for them and their children. She speaks from her heart, with a warm, honest, compelling voice of reason. She gets it right.
— Claire McCarthy, MD, FAAP
    Pediatrician and Medical Communications Editor, Boston Children's Hospital

—◦◊◦—

For Finn and Oden

Two little boys who endlessly inspire me

to improve the health of children everywhere.

I am hopelessly and forever your

loving, awestruck mom…

Table of Contents

Acknowledgments

I am seriously indebted to my Seattle Children's Hospital public relations and content advisor, Jennifer Seymour. Jennifer has championed my ideas, stood behind me amid tears and triumphs, and been a level sounding board over the years as I've evolved my thinking and my work. Like me, she believes in the power of technology to align doctors and patients. She and the team at Seattle Children's have been immensely helpful in changing the health communication space; David, Alyse, Mike, Louise, Craig, Mary, Scott, Diana, and Stacey's partnership throughout the duration of my writing and innovation career thus far has been immensely valuable.

I'm also so thankful for generous peers and ongoing mentors in the health and (social) media space, including Bryan Vartabedian, MD; Claire McCarthy, MD, FAAP; Natasha Burgert, MD, FAAP; Susannah Fox; Roni Zeiger, MD; Alex Drane; Dave Chase; Alanna Levine, MD, FAAP; Ari Brown, MD, FAAP; Jennifer Shu, MD, FAAP; Laura Jana, MD, FAAP; Tanya Altmann, MD, FAAP; Jordan Shlain, MD; Edgar Marcuse, MD, FAAP; Paul Offit, MD, FAAP; Kellie Cheadle; and Dave deBronkart. Their vision, courage, camaraderie, and friendship are sustaining. Additionally, there are tens of thousands of people to thank on Twitter. Thank you.

But it's my family who serves as my most trusted advisor. Each and every blog post I've written has been read by my husband, Jonathan, and my mom, Karen. My mom edits with a red pen just as she did when I was in the fifth grade but always sees the bigger landscape. You also have no idea how many times she's been with the boys "just 'another hour' so I can finish some writing." My husband, an academic, pediatric radiologist by day and fearless best friend by night, has lent days of advice gently, each and every step of the way. Amid all the noise I make in the world he continues with his steady, governed focus, his professionalism, and doing what is right for children and our boys with unparalleled and quiet leadership. He sees the long-term vision in this world. Without his support, his unrelenting commitment to my own work, and his belief in who I am and what I believe I can do to improve health care, I could never have maintained this momentum.

Having a partner like Jonathan is entirely the luxury of my life. Being welcomed, embraced, supported, and celebrated by his parents, Bill and Lois Swanson, is an auspicious joy. I'm one of those people who adores my in-laws.

I will also be forever indebted to beloved Cindini and the late Stephen Larson, MD. Dr Larson invited me into the profession of medicine when I was still a child. Without him I would never have known the potential of a career in medicine for making change and healing. The Larsons provided a literal and spiritual home for me at the end of my childhood. With selfless grace, they launched me into the real world. Every child deserves this generosity. Few get it.

Lastly, with a full heart, I must express my thanks to the patients and families who allow me into their lives at The Everett Clinic and the readers of the Seattle Mama Doc blog (www.seattlemamadoc.com) these past years. My gratitude is cavernous. Parents, physicians, children, innovators, marketers, teens, ethicists, psychologists, bloggers, dissenters, and supporters have all provided an incredible education for me. I am so thankful for people like Viki, Jen, Claire, Susannah, Carolyn, Paul, Mark, Fred, Katie, Emily, Kelly, Michele, Kathleen, Ed, Jay, Stacey, Susi, Evelyn, and Matt. I know you'll never know how much I count on you, but I'll keep trying to tell you. To those of you who courageously voice up, follow along, and help keep my feet planted firmly in my mission—you mean so much.

To those who believe the Internet and thousands of words in a book can save lives, let us sustain the energy to go forward and continue this work. All of our children depend on it.

Foreword

I have often bemoaned the fact that kids don't come with instruction manuals. There is no singular directive on how to raise a child, no primers on parenting before you head home from the hospital, babe in arms. The next best thing, of course, is a great pediatrician.

Before my son was born 10 years ago, my friends with children urged me to "interview" pediatricians. I had no idea that such a concept existed, but as a journalist, I was all for it. After making a few exploratory phone calls, I discovered that nearly every single pediatric office held evening meet and greets, a time for expectant parents to show up after hours to politely grill the doctors and hear their philosophies on taking care of children.

I ended up going with a practice in which the pediatricians weren't afraid to share their own adventures and misfortunes in child-rearing; in which they humanized the grand experiment of taking a 7-pound bundle and teaching it to eat, read, be kind to others, and clean up after themselves (the latter, in my home, is still a work in progress).

Wendy Sue Swanson, MD, MBE, FAAP, is that sort of pediatrician. She can quote research from medical journals with the most learned of practitioners, but she's also willing to bring those statistics to life. When I moved to the Pacific Northwest and began covering parenting and pediatrics, I kept running across her Seattle Mama Doc blog. It was chock-full of useful information delivered in candid, snappy prose, but it was also deeply thoughtful and insightful. From reading her posts, I felt like I knew her. And yet even though we lived in the same city, we hadn't met until research I was doing on vaccine-hesitant parents led me directly to her. Vaccine hesitancy is one of Wendy Sue's passions. At her practice, she's proud to be the pediatrician with the highest rate of vaccinated patients—not because she guilts parents or strong-arms them into immunizing but because she openly empathizes with their concerns.

The morning after actress Jenny McCarthy, a vocal opponent of vaccines, went on *Oprah* to say that vaccines had caused her son's autism, Wendy Sue saw a baby for her 1-year-old checkup. The baby's mom had seen the show, and she was terrified. Instead of brushing her off and deriding McCarthy, spouting statistics, or quoting policies, Wendy Sue listened. She nodded her head and looked the mom in the eye. Then she explained that research had unequivocally shown no association between vaccines and autism. She added that as a pediatrician who knows the research in and out, she fully vaccinates her own 2 children. What she didn't do was make that mom feel ignorant or crazy. Instead, she identified with her: "I think about those stories too when my kids got their shots," she told the mom. "I know the science, but I'm still a mom and I worry about my kids."

That honesty, combined with the facts about immunization, tipped the scales. The woman still wasn't thrilled about it, but she got her baby vaccinated because Wendy Sue had dared to share her own vulnerability as a mother.

It's that kind of openness and candor that infuses *Mama Doc Medicine: Finding Calm and Confidence in Parenting, Child Health, and Work-Life Balance.* There are essays on bacteria and bouncy houses, soft spots, separation anxiety, and—eek—lice. And because she's an ardent proponent of social media as a catalyst to improve health care, you'll find tweets interspersed in the content (along with recommendations for the best pediatric accounts on Twitter and Facebook), plus full-page infographics on important child health topics.

But mostly you'll find classic Wendy Sue—open, honest, funny, heartwarming, authoritative, and authentic. Just the kind of partner you'll want as you and your children navigate the maze that is childhood.

Bonnie Rochman

Bonnie Rochman is a health journalist who has written about parenting, pediatrics, and science for Time, The New York Times, The Wall Street Journal, *and* Scientific American.

Introduction

Loving Your Children More Than Imaginable: Modern Parenthood, a Blog, and a Mission for More

The thing that sweeps us all off our feet is the unexpected adoration, the insuppressible laughter, and the unconditional love we have for our children. Before children, boundless love seems possible. After we meet our children (however and wherever that happens), there's typically an immediate acknowledgment that parenthood exceeds our expectations. We often find ourselves gasping for clear air amid the ergonomics of daily life with our newborns and children. I learned quickly as a pediatrician and mom that parenting is a full-contact, full-time, and fully terrifying job.

Of course it's obvious that parenting is a rare flower and a thorny rose; it's not easy on the mind or body. Parts of parenthood are not only terrifying, they're exquisitely painful too. Our human vulnerability is heightened the day we begin to expect the arrival of a child.

When we're young, we learn that true love takes up huge real estate in our heart. When we become parents, we learn that the love for our children takes up even more.

I started to listen online long before I began to speak there. Officially, I started writing about parenthood and pediatrician-hood in fall 2009. The inertia to start writing and capturing thoughts using social tools came from my frustration with myths beginning to circulate widely online. The myths were predominately about the safety of vaccines, but mistruths also were creeping in about safe sleep, how to feed a baby, and the essentials of one parenting style over another. I heard stories about instinct, motherhood, and thimerosal misplaced and misaligned with the expertise that existed in copious research. I started to realize there were parents and pediatricians going against the grain—and parents were increasingly looking for insights on how to care for their children online. I knew I needed to speak out.

With the birth of my first son, Finn, in 2006 and my second son, Oden, in 2008, parenting became the focus of my life. Like my friends, I began to house more and more fearful anecdotes in my heart. I heard mistruths and scary stories. Even though I could deny their validity in my head, I often couldn't seem to shake the legacy of their power on my heart.

I was lucky; the science for prevention of pediatric disease was still safely in arm's reach for me because of my extensive training, my ongoing pediatric practice, and the incredible mentors from my medical education. Yet in practice, many parents told me they didn't have the same access to data or didn't hold the same value for science. As more and more messages were coming in from my Facebook feed, links in my inbox, and parents' concerns in the examination room, I knew I could sit on my hands only so long. I knew I had to ramp up my efforts to bring science to the forefront and join my friends, colleagues, families in clinic, and fellow physicians online in a more thoughtful, productive fashion.

My hope to do more jelled well with the social tools of our time. As a physician I feel I was born just at the right time.

In spring 2009, I approached Seattle Children's Hospital about teaming up to provide credible, evidence-based, passionate parenting information in real time. Rather than being a 10-second sound bite or 10 minutes or 10 days too late on the evening news, I proposed we could respond in real time, online. I could control the whole message and get the whole story out using a blog, a Twitter feed, and Facebook.

I wanted to share what it felt like to be a parent and pediatrician authentically. I wanted families to hear the "real story," not just what they were *supposed* to be told. I wanted to detail truths from new research with parents, doctors, and caregivers everywhere.

Seattle Children's Hospital and I settled on the concept of me authoring a blog, one that was entirely uncensored, organically conceived, and authentically delivered. At the time, David Perry was running the communications department at the hospital. He'd worked at Microsoft and Cranium prior to being at the hospital, so he clearly understood the frenetic flow of information that existed because of the Internet. Auspiciously, he also believed in my mission of doctoring outside the exam room. Someone once told me I'd get along with David because he spoke just as quickly as I did, but when I met him it was obvious that our mutual mission to improve the lives of children everywhere allowed us to come together quickly. He became a necessary champion for me. I started to blog my experience about parenthood, pediatric research, and unfolding parenting topics.

Four years and more than 400 blog posts later, Seattle Mama Doc (www.seattlemamadoc.com) continues to unfold on a weekly basis on the Seattle Children's Web site. Controversial parenting topics persist while new evidence is published in fire-hydrant fashion in medical journals. There is never a lack of topics to cover, and my boys serve up endless examples for sharing observations, insights, and pitfalls of parenting in modern times.

The messages captured here are an amalgamation of some of the most frequently read blog posts tossed together with some new ideas, new tips, and infographics to provide clarity. I'm thrilled to shine new light on some of this valuable data and so thankful that the American Academy of Pediatrics partnered with me to publish this book.

Of course the book is not just about science. Because I started blogging when both boys were younger than 3 years, I've also captured quite a bit of my struggle to maintain sanity and strive for balance in a very busy household. The work-life balance challenge exists for all working parents, and my hope is that my insights into the whole parenting-while-working ordeal will help you maintain a superior sense of calm. I've yet to find an easy solution to the discomfort that comes when we're parenting and working outside our homes, but there are so many glimpses of sincere joy amid the chaotic schedule that it's easy to keep iterating the fulcrum to make it better and better. Each and every day my boys grow, I realize we have a different, demanding job.

WendySueSwanson MD @SeattleMamaDoc

The moment you realize your children remember everything is also the moment you reconnect w the reality that parenting is a high-stakes job

Part 1

Prevention

KEEPING CALM ABOUT CRYING

Every infant cries; it's a part of being a baby. Yet crying still puts many of us on edge; it's simply instinctive to want to make it go away. It's important to know the big range of normal and when there might be a concern.

THE BIG NORMAL

"Unsoothable" crying represents **5% to 15%** of all infant restlessne

Infants cry increasingly from **2 WEEKS** of age, peaking at **6 TO 8 WEEKS**

Dramatically improves af **~3 TO 4 MONTHS** of age

Most babies cry unpredictably, resistant to our best efforts to comfort.

Babies tend to cry most in the evening, wh we're all exhausted and run down.

Even normal, healthy babies may cry for long periods—an hour or more—and may appear to be in pain.

COULD IT BE COLIC?

Colic has traditionally been defined using the rule of 3s.

DOES YOUR INFANT CRY

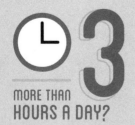

3
MORE THAN
HOURS A DAY?

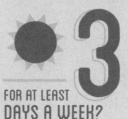

3
FOR AT LEAST
DAYS A WEEK?

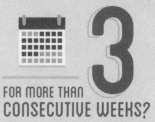

3
FOR MORE THAN
CONSECUTIVE WEEKS?

Although the rule of 3s can help families define it, ultimately the label of "colic" doesn't stop the crying.

WHAT SHOULD YOU DO?

DON'T BE TEMPTED TO REACH FOR MEDICATIONS OR CURES.

A 2011 *Pediatrics* article evaluated 15 large studies (including nearly 1,000 babies) to determine the efficacy of things like

Sugary/glucose solutions	Infant massage	Probiotics	Herbal supplements	Chiropractor's manipulation

THE RESULTS?

NONE OF THESE MEASURABLY HELP CRYING.

THE FOLLOWING 3-STEP ACTION PLAN, THOUGH, IS GREAT FOR A FUSSY INFANT:

1. Walk, talk, and soothe your baby in ways she loves.

2. If crying continues, know that it's natural to feel frustrated. It's always OK to place your baby in the crib and take a short break.

3. If you feel frustrated or angry, place your baby in the crib on her back and step away. Take turns with your partner. Never shake a baby!

SOURCES
- www.pediatrics.org/content/127/4/720.full
- www.purplecrying.info/what-is-the-period-of-purple-crying.php

Part 1
Prevention

Introduction

Many pediatricians commend themselves on doing the least. We love to be the physician who prescribes the least antibiotics, orders the fewest computed tomography scans, and helps our patients avoid emergency department visits the most. We want children to thrive without causing unnecessary harm. A big part of being a comprehensive pediatrician is helping families know where research resides to prevent disease.

Often, when we intervene the least, we preserve health the most. Knowing the wide range of normal takes expertise coupled with experience. This is not to say it's a lack of attention pediatricians seek; it's just we want focused attention to know when not to poke around and do more.

Parents, of course, want the same thing.

The resilience of childhood health is astounding. As parents, our job is to provide the best setup. We want to layer prevention efforts to afford our children the least suffering, pain, and illness. We want to feel like we've done our very best. We want to tuck away any guilt that nags at us too.

Part 1, Prevention, showcases recent research and marries experience in the office and online spaces to provide snippets and ideas for you to protect your children and set them up to thrive. From a lice infestation, to tips on buying the right sunscreen, to a colicky baby, to watching too much television, may you step forward knowing you are doing this one right.

1

Science of the Soft Spot

The soft spot on the top of my baby's head was one of my favorite places to run my hand. I don't know why exactly, but it seemed one of those places on him that truly represented his babyhood. One way I knew that his infancy wasn't quite gone and my baby days weren't over yet. When Oden turned 1 year of age and I started to feel the dread of his baby-ness slipping through my fingers, I kept mentioning the soft spot to my patients when they would ask about him. I was hoping it would somehow prolong the period of infancy and I wouldn't have to wake up and find myself with 2 grown boys in the house.

The emotional yo-yo between pure excitement about them growing up with the simultaneous dread of losing these baby moments remains real and palpable. The essence of parenthood, I suppose, is that stew of anxiety-thrill-dread-adoration-excitement as the days unfold and you hope for new things for your little baby while lamenting the loss of precious moments of who your baby is on a Monday in January. The soft spot was always a good place to go to calm my inner anxiety about my toddlers walking out the door to college.

> *The emotional yo-yo between pure excitement about them growing up with the simultaneous dread of losing these baby moments remains real and palpable.*

Lots of new parents ask me about caring for the soft spot. As the first year unfolds, it is the soft spot (aka, fontanelle) in the front/top portion of a baby's head that parents ask about—the anterior fontanelle. I think we all conjure up crazy worries about an errant flying pencil landing in it. Or pushing too hard and squishing something important. I've never experienced, read, or heard of this happening.

Science About the Soft Spot

- Infants are born with about 6 soft spots in their heads to allow for the big squeeze through the birth canal.
- In general, pediatricians and parents can only feel 2 soft spots at birth (one in the front portion of the skull and one in the back of the head on top). Even then, we can usually only feel one spot after a baby is about 1 month of age—the anterior fontanelle.
- Ninety percent of soft spots (anterior fontanelle) close between about 7 and 19 months of age.

The soft spot is often a diamond shape. But it doesn't always feel like that, and soft spots vary in size dramatically from one baby to the next. It can be anywhere from a couple inches across to just fingertip size.

I think we're all curious (pediatricians, parents, relatives, neighbors, the lady at the grocery store who touches your baby before you have time to stop her) about the soft spot as it reflects a tender spot on our baby. A reflection of all that growth and potential housed in one little head. You're not alone if you find yourself thinking/worrying about the soft spot at 2:00 am. When Oden was born, I asked his pediatrician at 2 separate visits to reassure me about his soft spot. It just felt big! I think she thought I was crazy. I remember feeling embarrassed to bring it up (thinking she would think I should know better) even though I was worried about it. She reassured me. He was growing well, his head was growing well, and he was doing what he was supposed to do. Kelly Evans, MD, FAAP, a friend and pediatrician who specializes in craniofacial pediatrics (head and face), said she too asked about her son's soft spot after he was born and worried like so many other moms.

Your pediatrician will always look at your baby's head growth and the size of the soft spot at checkups. Only rarely do pediatricians send patients to see craniofacial experts. When Dr Evans sees patients in the craniofacial clinic for evaluation of the soft spot, the craniofacial team doesn't just look at the soft spot; they feel and evaluate the spot in the context of the baby. "Our opinion of the soft spot all comes in context of their head shape, their developmental skills, and OFC (measurement around the head). I am never just looking at the fontanelle alone but how the baby's head is growing and how it looks and feels. And how they act when we examine them." Although we talk a lot about this spot, it doesn't often represent a health problem. More often, it's a true reflection of health.

More Science to Calm You About That Soft Spot

- The fontanelle or soft spot at the front of a baby's head is the intersection of 4 bones (2 frontal and 2 parietal) in the skull.
- The anterior fontanelle is not fragile but also not the spot you truly want to expose to the elements. It's soft and vulnerable as there is no bone between your baby's brain and the outside world. Good planning in the anatomy world afforded multiple layers of tough tissue protecting your baby at that spot.
- The soft spot serves a dual purpose for your baby—it allows for your baby's fast-growing brain to expand and also provides an elastic-like cushion to the skull until it ultimately closes.
- When a baby transitions from infant to toddler and starts walking (falling!), that fibrous area allows for the bones to shift and absorb impact on a fall.
- You'll sometimes see the soft spot pulse a bit as you watch blood flow around your baby's brain and skull when she is calm and resting.

When it comes to the soft spot, the reality is just to be gentle and smart and trust your instincts. And watch out for those flying pencils.

Take a peek at a 3-D reconstruction of a computed tomography scan of a patient's skull showing that diamond-shaped fontanelle over the forehead area. (For more, see the video at http://bit.ly/mdm-3DCT.)

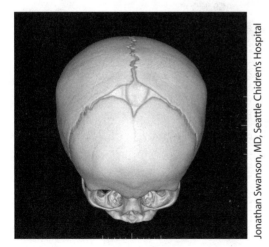

Jonathan Swanson, MD, Seattle Children's Hospital

Mama Doc Vitals

Fact: Ninety percent of soft spots close sometime between 9 and 19 months.

Size and Shape: Most soft spots really vary in size. Try not to compare one baby with another. In general, soft spots are diamond shaped and between the size of the circle of a soda can to the size of your fingertip.

Check out this graph from the only study of its kind (in 1949!) regarding the timing of soft spot closures in infants.

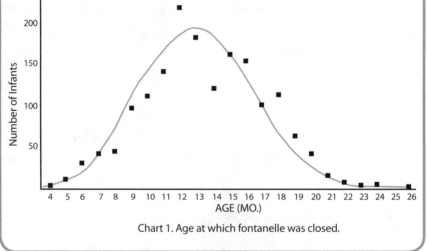

Chart 1. Age at which fontanelle was closed.

Source: Aisenson MR. Closing of the anterior fontanelle. *Pediatrics*. 1950;6(2):223–226

2

A Spoonful of Bacteria for Baby?

I'm becoming more of a believer in giving children probiotics. Not for everything and not for everyone; I really don't think we should put them in the water. Probiotics, essentially live, "good" bacteria we use to supplement our diet (usually *Lactobacillus acidophilus* in the United States), are becoming more available and recommended by more physicians. The role microbes play in our health is a hot topic. Probiotics are thought to improve intestinal health by restoring/elevating levels of helpful bacteria while concurrently diminishing the population of harmful ones. Bacteria in the intestine are a normal part of our digestive health, but population counts of bacteria living in our gut may be altered by illness, antibiotic use, ingested/modified foods, or life circumstance. What we eat and where we travel to drink water change what lives in our gut. Research also finds that which bacteria cohabitate in our bodies may affect other illnesses outside the gut like eczema, allergies, or asthma.

In children, probiotic supplements may promote recovery from acute diarrhea by decreasing the number of episodes of diarrhea and the number of days. Studies find that if a child takes a probiotic while she is ill, that child will have about 1 less day of diarrhea from an illness and 1 to 2 less episodes of diarrhea starting 2 days later. Probiotics also may help prevent the development of diarrhea when children are taking antibiotics.

The reality is that many decisions we make affect our populations of bacteria. This starts on the day of birth. We know, for example, that babies born by cesarean delivery have different populations of bacteria in their poop when compared with those babies born vaginally, within a week after birth. So from the very beginning, the choices we make (or our parents make) may change the environment in our bodies. This ultimately may change our wellness.

Probiotics are often found naturally in food (yogurt with active cultures), while some yogurt and commercially available foods (and infant formula) are fortified with additional cultures. You can also buy *Lactobacillus* capsules (or other probiotics) at drugstores and health food stores. How active and how plentiful the probiotics remain in these products is up for debate. Probiotic supplements (and culture-fortified foods) are not regulated by the US Food and Drug Administration. How much is in a capsule or packet is unknown and likely inconsistent from brand to brand or day to day. And if the probiotic cultures are dead, they may do very little to promote change in your body. As a consumer, knowing whether a supplement is alive is impossible.

That being said, although the choices of probiotics are limited in the United States, the literature and research surrounding the alteration of a child's bacteria to preserve his health and wellness are fascinating and promising. Outside of *Lactobacillus*, relatively few studies have been done with US children and probiotics. But we're learning a lot from our European colleagues. The risks of giving a probiotic supplement continue to prove to be very low in children with a healthy immune system. But like anything in pediatrics, there is always theoretic risk when you intervene. A study by a set of doctors on the effect of probiotics on colicky babies may help us understand benefits early in life.

A 2010 Italian study evaluated the benefit of probiotics for fussy or colicky babies. Researchers found positive results in breastfed babies receiving daily probiotics called *Lactobacillus reuteri*. In Europe, probiotics are more carefully regulated than they are here in the United States, so it's possible this study really isn't applicable to our babies because we don't have access to the same supplements. In the study

- Colic was defined using the *rule of 3s*. A colicky baby is defined as *one younger than 3 months who cries more than 3 hours a day, more than 3 days a week, for at least 3 weeks.*
- About 50 exclusively breastfed colicky babies were randomized into 2 groups. One group of babies was fed a placebo/inert supplement with no probiotics, while the other group got *Lactobacillus* daily. Parents and researchers didn't know which babies got the bacteria (double-blind study).
- Among colicky babies who received the probiotic, there was a significant reduction in daily crying time at the end of the study (day 21) compared with the placebo group.
- Crying improved by the end of the study in both groups, as is expected with colic.
- Researchers also analyzed the poop from both sets of babies and found different bacterial populations between the groups of babies. Those given the probiotic had far more *Lactobacillus* in their stool.
- Researchers theorize that changes in intestinal environment (bacteria, ammonia) may have changed sensory experience for babies and thus their crying behaviors.

It's hard to prove that the bacteria fed to these babies is directly responsible for crying improvement, but significant differences in the 2 groups were noted. And although it may seem counterintuitive to families to feed their child bacteria, after we discuss benefits, many parents opt to supplement their children with *Lactobacillus* because of low cost and ease of administration (it can be sprinkled in anything). If your baby is a crier and you think and worry about colic, you may want to talk with your pediatrician about starting a *Lactobacillus* supplement. With the low risk, an improvement in crying would be good for everyone. The bottom line is that I don't think probiotics will cause a fussy baby any harm, and this is new research that indicates it may really help. A spoonful of bacteria for baby, then.

Mama Doc Vitals

Fact: Babies born vaginally are coated with microbes from their mothers' birth canals. Babies born by cesarean delivery are covered in microbes typically found on the skin of adults.

Supplements: Probiotics are available over the counter and come in packets, capsules, and powder form. You can open up capsules and sprinkle them over soft food or place into a bottle of pumped breast milk or formula.

Study: *Lactobacillus* is safe and effective as a treatment for children with acute infectious diarrhea: http://bit.ly/mdm-probiotics.

3

Mix and Match: Goldilocks Formula

Often new parents are nervous about mixing and matching the infant formula they offer their babies. They worry if they switch from one formula brand to another, they may cause their baby fussiness, stool changes, upset, or worse—they could put their baby at risk.

It's safe to mix and match infant formulas if you are following standard mixing instructions. Really.

Although spitting up or gassiness is usually not caused by the protein in formula (protein source is the big difference between cow's milk versus soy versus hypoallergenic formula), sometimes changing formula helps new babies and their parents who worry. Switching them up can even help clarify worries in some scenarios when a parent worries about excessive gassiness, intolerance, or significant "urping" or spitting up.

Experimentation with formula brands in an otherwise healthy newborn is OK. But it's not necessary at all, either.

It's fine to make a bottle that is half formula from the blue can and half formula from the yellow one. Fine to serve Similac one week, Enfamil the next, then Earth's Best or Good Start, followed by any other formula the following day. Fine to buy one brand that's on sale only to buy the other brand next week.

> *Experimentation with formula brands in an otherwise healthy newborn is OK. But it's not necessary at all, either.*

However, all this being said, I usually recommend that families don't switch often. Let time unfold and give your baby a chance to settle in. Don't react to every single poop. Give your baby a week or two on a formula before you give up or reach for a new can.

One of my best friends was unable to breastfeed and found that when she served her baby organic formula, he got constipated, but when she used non-organic, he didn't. She was determined to provide him as much organic food as possible but really hated seeing him strain to poop.

This is where the Goldilocks concept comes in—the goal of making things close to perfect or "just right." My friend texted me one night assuming that she couldn't mix and match formulas but "just wanted to check and see." I felt she could. Voilà! She found that making the "just-right" formula (half organic mixed with half conventional) provided a bit more balance for her newborn son. She found that when she fed him the "Goldilocks" bottle, the hard stools and potential constipation improved.

Fine by baby. Fine by pediatrician. Mama Bear felt better too.

Parents often want to buy the formula on sale; they wonder if they can switch it up and save money. I say yes. There is no danger in providing your baby differing formulas from one day to the next.

Think of it this way: babies who are breastfed have a slightly different milk each and every meal due to mom's variant diet. Although fat, calories, and protein count remain constant, flavor and variety changes. A slightly different recipe at every feed.

Goldilocks Infant Formula Rules

- Never add sugar, juice, or cow's milk to infant formula.
- Don't fix what isn't broken. No need to switch formula if you have no concerns.
- Don't dilute or concentrate the formula you make for your baby. Standard powdered formulas usually mix 1 scoop to every 2 ounces of water. Follow directions and use the scooper that comes with the formula.
- In the United States, in my opinion, it's safe to use tap water to mix infant formula. However, some families may want to avoid excess fluoride consumption from tap water for babies exclusively fed formula. Information from the Centers for Disease Control and Prevention on fluoride for formula feeders states that there is no need to purchase distilled water (in plastic bottles) and no reason to boil water prior to mixing; however, if you want, you can remove fluoride with a reverse osmosis filter system.
- If your baby is super-cranky or doesn't react well to a change in the formula you offer, or if you're worried about a potential intolerance or allergy, talk with your pediatrician about a plan for selecting the best infant formula for your baby.

- Continue to feed infant formula until your baby is 12 months of age. No Goldilocks mixing with cow's milk or other milk substitutes prior to that first birthday.

The Skinny on Formula

The American Academy of Pediatrics has adapted content from the popular book *Caring for Your Baby and Young Child: Birth to Age 5* and its HealthyChildren.org Web site on formula. Take a look!

To maintain safety standards for newborn and infant health in this country, an act of Congress governs the contents of infant formula, and the US Food and Drug Administration monitors all formulas. When shopping for infant formula, you'll find several basic types.

Cow's Milk–Based Formulas

- Most common type of formula sold.

- Made from cow's milk that has been dramatically changed to make it safe and more digestible. It is formulated to include the nutrients (as close to human milk as possible) newborns and infants need for healthy growth and development.

- The American Academy of Pediatrics (AAP) currently recommends that iron-fortified formula be used for all newborns and infants who are not breastfed or who are only partially breastfed, from birth to 1 year of age. Some mothers worry about the iron in infant formula causing constipation, but the amount of iron provided in infant formula does not contribute to constipation in babies.

- Most formulas also have docosahexaenoic acid (DHA) and arachidonic acid (AA) added to them, which are fatty acids, believed to be important for the development of a baby's brain and eyes.

Hydrolyzed Formulas (Hypoallergenic Formulas)

- They often are called *predigested,* meaning that their protein content has already been broken down into smaller proteins that can be digested more easily.

- In newborns and infants who have a high risk of developing allergies (eg, family history) and who have not been breastfed exclusively for 4 to 6 months, there is some evidence that skin conditions like eczema or atopic dermatitis can be prevented or delayed by feeding them extensively or partially hydrolyzed (hypoallergenic) formulas.

- Will help at least 90% of babies who have food allergies, which can cause symptoms such as hives, a runny nose, and intestinal problems.

- Tend to be costlier than regular formulas, so I recommend you only purchase them if necessary.

Soy Formulas

- Contain a protein (soy) and carbohydrate (glucose or sucrose) different from milk-based formulas.

- Sometimes recommended for babies unable to digest lactose, although simple lactose-free cow's milk–based formula is also available. Many newborns and infants have brief periods when they cannot digest lactose, particularly following bouts of diarrhea, which can damage the digestive enzymes in the lining of the intestines. But this is usually only a temporary problem and does not require a change in your baby's diet.

- It is rare for babies to have a significant problem digesting and absorbing lactose (although it tends to occur in older children and adults). If your pediatrician suggests a lactose-free formula, know that it provides your baby with everything that she needs to grow and develop just as a lactose-containing formula does.

- Not a good alternative when a true milk allergy is present because as many as half the babies who have milk allergy are also sensitive to soy protein.

- Some strict vegetarian parents choose to use soy formula because it contains no animal products. Remember that breastfeeding is the best option for vegetarian families.

- There is no evidence to support its effectiveness to prevent or ease the symptoms of colic or fussiness.

- The AAP believes that there are few circumstances in which soy formula should be chosen instead of cow's milk–based formula in term newborns and infants. One of these situations is in babies with a rare disorder called galactosemia.

Specialized Formulas

- Manufactured for babies with specific disorders or diseases. There are also formulas made specifically for premature babies.

- If your pediatrician recommends a specialized formula for your baby, follow the pediatrician's guidance about feeding requirements (eg, amounts, scheduling, special preparations) because it may be quite different from regular formulas.

- Some formulas also are fortified with probiotics, which are types of "friendly" bacteria. Others are now fortified with prebiotics, natural food substances that promote healthy intestinal lining.

Mama Doc Vitals

Bottom Line: It is totally OK to mix and match formulas, but remember—don't fix what isn't broken! No need to run experiments at home on formula if your baby is doing great.

Centers for Disease Control and Prevention Information on Water and Fluoride: http://bit.ly/mdm-fluoride

Infant Formula Information From MedlinePlus: http://bit.ly/mdm-formulas

Tip: If your baby is exclusively consuming infant formula reconstituted with fluoridated water, there may be an increased chance of mild dental fluorosis. To lessen this chance, you can use low-fluoride bottled water here and there when mixing infant formula.

At the Store: *Fluoride-Free Water:* Bottled water that is labeled as *deionized, purified, demineralized,* or *distilled* is fluoride free.

Colic, Crying, and the Period of
PURPLE Crying

Every infant cries. It's a part of being a baby, yet crying still puts many of us on edge. As parents, we want to calm our babies and prevent crying; it's simply instinctive to want to make it go away. The period of time when our babies cry most (between 1 and 2 months of age) can be entirely exhausting, unsettling, and unnerving. As we transition into parenthood, one of the most difficult challenges can be learning to soothe our crying babies. One expert, Ronald Barr, MA, MDCM, FRCPC, refers to this period of crying as the PURPLE period. I'll explain the PURPLE period, but first let's talk a bit about colic, news today about using alternative "folk" treatments, and ultimately what it may mean when someone, a doctor or not, tells you that you've got a "colicky" baby.

A 2011 *Pediatrics* article evaluated 15 large studies (including nearly 1,000 babies) to determine if things like infant massage, probiotics, chiropractor's manipulation, herbal supplements, and sugary/glucose solutions really helped

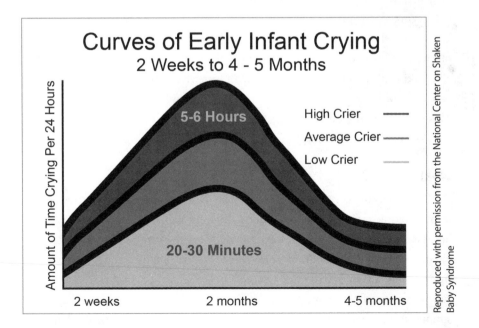

Curves of Early Infant Crying
2 Weeks to 4 - 5 Months

Amount of Time Crying Per 24 Hours

5-6 Hours

High Crier
Average Crier
Low Crier

20-30 Minutes

2 weeks   2 months   4-5 months

Reproduced with permission from the National Center on Shaken Baby Syndrome "colicky" babies stop crying. The results proved unfortunate. *None of these interventions helped infants who were crying/fussy/screaming their heads off.*

Two things to think about with these findings: first, when you're frustrated with a baby's fussing/crying, don't reach for these remedies as solutions or cure-alls. As we know now, there's not a lot of evidence to use any of these remedies. Secondly, don't confuse the word "natural" with "harmless" or "safe." Many of these herbal and complementary remedies come with labels that say "natural." Natural doesn't confer safety. A limitation of interpreting data from the 15 studies reviewed was the reality that little time was spent reporting side effects to interventions and therapeutics. It may simply be because there were few, but researchers are unsure.

We only want to use medications in infants that prove effective.

WendySueSwanson MD @SeattleMamaDoc

No evidence massage, herbal supps, sugar solutions, chiropractors, or probiotics improve infant cry/"colic" symptoms
http://bit.ly/hQdQjK

The most important thing to do for a fussy infant is to find ways for you to soothe your baby. But know that you won't always be successful. If your baby has been fed, burped, and changed; is warm and comfortably dressed; and is still crying, don't spend all of your energy determining the why behind the cry. Unfortunately, you likely won't find the answer! Rather, spend time figuring out what helps—things like rocking, holding, walking outside, taking a stroller ride, taking a car ride, running a faucet of water for white noise, changing your baby's position, or putting baby down for a break in her crib. Breaks are key. This space can provide a break for both of you. What's most important is that you, as a caregiver, find soothing in times of stress too!

What Is Colic?

Oddly, diagnosing colic can be controversial. Not every pediatrician uses the term. Infantile crying is expected and varies from baby to baby. The key point here is that *all babies cry.* From the moment they are born, babies have their first big important cry to clear fluid from their lungs. Crying time starts to accelerate from 2 weeks of age with a peak around 6 to 8 weeks, then ultimately dramatically improves after about 3 to 4 months of age. By definition, colic goes away simply with time. But not all babies are alike; some cry far more than others.

- Colic has traditionally been defined using the rule of 3s; that is, infants who cry more than 3 hours a day, at least 3 days a week, for more than 3 consecutive weeks. However, the cutoff of 3 hours is entirely arbitrary. Although the rule of 3s can help families define it, ultimately the label of colic doesn't solve the frustrating crying. As any parent can attest, 2 hours and 59 minutes of crying versus 3 hours and 10 minutes of crying a day certainly isn't very different. So defining colic is only a part of it. Sometimes, though, I think parents feel better having a label to the crying, a name to help define it. It gives them scope for their struggles and frustrations. But having a diagnosis of colic doesn't mean there is something wrong with your baby.
- Infantile crying is common and variable, with some studies finding nearly 20% or more of babies demonstrating "excessive" crying every week. It's hard to define what is normal and what is abnormal, hence the controversy in colic's definition. Often how we experience our infant's crying varies from parent to parent too, which again confuses the labeling.
- Most parents and pediatricians think of colic as crying that is more intense, is difficult to soothe or resistant to soothing, and lasts for long periods of time. Dr Barr, an expert on infant crying, told me that roughly speaking, "unsoothable" crying represents about 5% to 15% of all crying and fussing that infants do. The rest is made up by "fussing" (about 65%) and "crying" (about 35%).
- *Excessive crying can be seen in all babies, no matter if they are breastfed or formula fed, first or second born, boy or girl, or premature or full term.*

Crying can be extremely difficult on caregivers, particularly because crying peaks in the late afternoon and evening when parents are already exhausted. This is a huge part of the diagnosis and a huge part of the therapy. Recognizing the toll on caregivers is essential for supporting the baby.

Is It Just Infants Who Have "Colic" and Excessive Crying?

Yes, again, crying is a part of every new baby's life but varies dramatically between one baby and another and even between siblings. Just like weight and height vary, crying varies dramatically between one healthy baby and another.

Do We Know What Causes Colic?

The short answer: No. Not knowing for sure what causes excessive crying and colic is part of the problem with helping families understand that testing (blood work or radiology studies) and medication interventions are overwhelmingly not needed. However, theories about colic and excessive crying look to food allergies, formula intolerance, gas formation, and intestinal cramping. Many researchers believe crying is a normal part of an infant's life and that the "painful" look on their face or sound of their cry may not represent a medical problem but rather a spectrum of normal infant crying.

> Some babies may have high amounts of normal crying that are exacerbated by illness or cause. This could be a sensitivity to cow's milk protein (dairy), excessive gas, or an intolerance to formula or other proteins. If you think your baby is fussy in a typical pattern, acutely changes in the way he cries, or cries only with feeding, it's absolutely something to share with your pediatrician.

We know that lots of other species, mammals, and even non-primates who breastfeed have similar trends of rising distress or crying in the first few months of life. Some researchers theorize the why behind all this crying lies in evolutionary terms—babies who cry are cared for, form attachments and better bonds with caregivers and parents, and are more likely to be picked up, held, and protected from predators.

What Is the Period of PURPLE Crying?

PURPLE is an acronym to help define the normal pattern of crying for babies. It describes typical crying behaviors. Again, all babies cry with a **P**eak in the minutes or hours of daily crying around 6 to 8 weeks after birth. Most babies will cry **U**npredictably (unprovoked or unexpectedly), and their cries will be **R**esistant to the best of our efforts to comfort. Many normal, healthy babies will cry and it will look like they are in **P**ain and will cry for **L**ong periods (up to an hour or more). And finally, they tend to cry most in the **E**vening when we're all exhausted and run down.

Sometimes just knowing the range of normal can help us calm down. The most important thing for our babies is that we take care of ourselves too, in our frustrations to soothe crying. Taking breaks and taking turns caring for babies

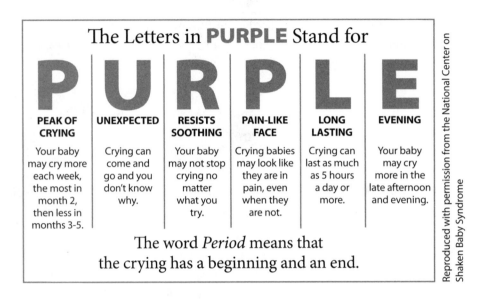

The Letters in **PURPLE** Stand for

P	U	R	P	L	E
PEAK OF CRYING	**UNEXPECTED**	**RESISTS SOOTHING**	**PAIN-LIKE FACE**	**LONG LASTING**	**EVENING**
Your baby may cry more each week, the most in month 2, then less in months 3-5.	Crying can come and go and you don't know why.	Your baby may not stop crying no matter what you try.	Crying babies may look like they are in pain, even when they are not.	Crying can last as much as 5 hours a day or more.	Your baby may cry more in the late afternoon and evening.

The word *Period* means that
the crying has a beginning and an end.

when you get frustrated can be essential. Talk with your partners, nannies, or any other caregivers about the PURPLE period so they too know what to expect.

What Can You Do to Treat Colic?

Time, support for parents and caregivers, and partnerships with pediatricians are essential. Sometimes, having a baby evaluated for allergies or intolerance is part of the workup to define additional treatments, but not in the majority of infants. Sometimes modifying a breastfeeding mom's diet (restricting dairy, usually) can help and is worth a try. When you're worried about your baby, call the pediatrician, visit with him or her, and discuss your concerns and what your plans are to soothe and support your crying baby.

Most important in treating infantile crying is treating parents' frustrations and giving them tools to HELP learn to soothe their baby! Many of my friends and patients have enjoyed reading and watching *The Happiest Baby on the Block* book and DVD by Harvey Karp, MD, FAAP, because it gives them a set of tools to try to soothe their baby's cries.

We know that excessive crying is a risk factor for child abuse and shaking of infants. In fact, the number one most common trigger for a baby to be shaken is inconsolable crying.

We know that in times of stress, shaking of infants is higher than usual. Helping families find support and an action plan for crying is most important, particularly because crying in infants is self-limited, meaning it gets better simply with time. Sometimes it's hard for us to wait when we're exhausted and overwhelmed. It's OK to ask for help, even if it means seeing the pediatrician every week or more if needed.

> *The number one most common trigger for a baby to be shaken is inconsolable crying.*

How to Cope With Colic or Fussy Infants

Infantile colic is difficult to treat, but the great news is it goes away with time! The majority of excessive crying stops around 3 months of age. Talk with your pediatrician about your concerns so together you can develop a plan on communicating about crying or evaluating potential causes of crying. If your baby's cries seem to mimic the PURPLE period, resist spending time figuring out what makes a baby cry (you won't figure it out) and spend energy putting in place plans for soothing, supports for you and your spouse, enlisting evening care from friends and family, respite care for you, and finding techniques to successfully deal with crying and soothing babies.

The following 3-step action plan is great for helping a fussy infant:

1. Walk, talk, and comfort your baby. *Go outside* where crying isn't as loud and you can be relieved by space. This often helps comfort baby and stop the crying. The fresh air and break from all the noise inside will help you too.
2. If crying goes on a long time and parent/caregiver is frustrated, it's OK to *walk away* for a period. Put baby in the crib on her back or in the bassinet and take a break for 10 to 15 minutes. Have a soft drink, grab your phone, walk outside, or sit on your porch. Take a break! Your baby will be fine and you'll do better and have more energy when returning to your baby's cries.
3. Never shake a baby. She won't stop crying and it can have serious or even deadly results. Harming or hitting a baby will never curb crying. And know with ongoing gentle comforting, holding, and soothing, you can never spoil an infant! All that love will only help support your bond with your baby.

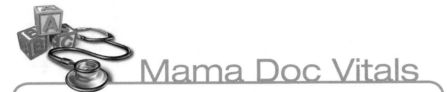

Mama Doc Vitals

Fact: All babies cry. Quieter babies who cry only a few minutes a day don't have "better" parents; they just have lucky ones.

Tip: Colic and infantile crying generally improve after 3 months of age, with 60% of excessive crying resolving by 3 months!

Medications: No medications have been proven to cure fussiness in babies. If you're concerned about your baby, don't hesitate to go in to see the doctor.

Study: Complementary medicines and massage for infant colic: http://bit.ly/mdm-colic

Reading a Growth Chart

When you go to the pediatrician for a well-child check, you'll always review your baby's or child's growth. It's probably the most important piece of data your pediatrician gets. The reason is, it can capture so much about your child's vitality.

In the first 3 years, we use one growth chart that looks at the head's circumference and the weight and length. It's based on gender and lots of data. We watch for changes in the size of head circumference in infancy because we want to know that the brain is growing. Growth grids have been used since the 1970s, but back in 2000, they were revised to really reflect different cultural and ethnic diversities that exist within our population.

What we want from a growth grid is to really map out the ideal growth for children. This isn't like grades in school. *When your child comes in at the 10th percentile, it's really no better or worse than coming in at the 90th.* What we care about most is the trend at which your baby or child gains weight, height, or head circumference.

After age 2, you can use the growth chart to expand between the ages of 2 and 20. In addition to weight and height at that point, we also look at body mass index, that number where we try to capture how children's proportionality is. Are they at risk for overweight or are they too lean?

Everything from genetics, to environment, to nutrition, to activity, to health problems really influence how your child grows. Why we review it each time is to talk about threats to your baby's or child's health and ways that you can take great opportunity to make changes.

When you're looking at a growth grid, what you want to focus on is how your child is changing. One static point on the growth grid isn't as relevant as 5 data points over time. You want to know rates at which your baby or child is growing and the rate compared with the grid.

As you follow the grid along from infancy into toddlerhood, you'll notice that each time it will rise. Each data point at each set of time will increase. We care about the rate at which your baby or child grows, not the number.

Parents often come in to the office and say, "What percent is she at?" She might be at the 13th percentile; that might be phenomenal based on where she's been previously, or it might be concerning. Don't focus on the number. Have your pediatrician, family doctor, or nurse practitioner help you understand what the trends are for your baby's growth.

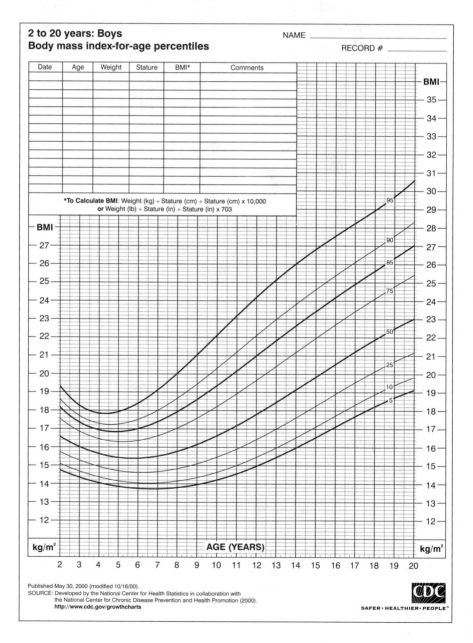

2 to 20 years: Boys
Body mass index-for-age percentiles

NAME _____

RECORD # _____

*To Calculate BMI: Weight (kg) ÷ Stature (cm) ÷ Stature (cm) x 10,000
or Weight (lb) ÷ Stature (in) ÷ Stature (in) x 703

Published May 30, 2000 (modified 10/16/00).
SOURCE: Developed by the National Center for Health Statistics in collaboration with
the National Center for Chronic Disease Prevention and Health Promotion (2000).
http://www.cdc.gov/growthcharts

SAFER · HEALTHIER · PEOPLE™

> *If your doctor doesn't have a computer in the examination room, ask to see the chart on paper or on a computer in the office.*

Parents, pediatricians, and nurses have been using growth charts since the late 1970s to track growth in infants and children. The charts were revised back in 2000 as data for the first charts (from a small study in Ohio) didn't accurately reflect the cultural and ethnic diversity of our communities.

The hallmark of a well-child check is the review of a child's growth. Growth can be a reflection of a child's overall health, nutrition, or tolerance of possible underlying medical conditions. So understanding what your doctor or nurse practitioner says about your child's growth should be a priority.

If your doctor doesn't have a computer in the examination room, ask to see the chart on paper or on a computer in the office. It will not only inform you, I suspect it will delight you to see what your child has done since the last time he was seen.

The human body really is a fine-tuned machine, and growth is simply astounding if you really stop to think of it. It's true your baby will at least double his weight by 6 months and triple it by about 1 year of age.

If you have a challenge understanding how your child is growing or how the growth chart is presented, demand clarification. It's OK if you don't understand the presentation of facts on these grids; have confidence to speak up and ask the doctor or nurse practitioner to explain it.

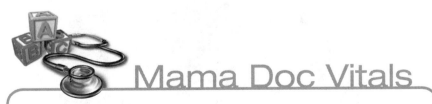

Mama Doc Vitals

Video: Watch this video in which I explain how to read a growth chart: http://bit.ly/mdm-GCvideo.

Perspective: A reminder that nothing is "better" about a child who's at 85% compared to 15% on the height grid. Both are the same distance from average!

Links: Centers for Disease Control and Prevention growth charts: http://bit.ly/mdm-GrowthCharts

KidsHealth Growth Charts: http://bit.ly/mdm-GrowthChartInfo

6

100 Calories

I often talk about how any food packaged in boxes or bags with red/orange/yellow spectrum of the rainbow detailing will lure you into eating more—in fact, studies prove it. Think about it—think fast food, junk food, and candy. So much of the packaging of the junk is designed to stimulate hunger (those red-orange-yellow colors do just that). To help us deal with this color lure, I like to mention one great 2010 study that may change your world.

Think about calories as weights in a balance. Keeping the balance of what goes in and what is used up is essential. And every 100 calories of red-orange-yellow packaged goods can make a difference, especially if you have a child living in your house. If you acknowledge the finding that about 1 out of every 4 children between the ages of 4 and 8 years eats fast food on a typical day, this has relevance to at least about a quarter of us, every single day.

A 2010 study published in *Pediatrics* found that when parents are aware of the calorie count in McDonald's fast-food items, they order less-caloric foods for their preschoolers (aged 3–6 years). In a Seattle pediatric clinic, about 100 parents filled out McDonald's menu choices for lunch for themselves and their preschooler. Families who had menus that included calorie content for each item listed selected meals that were about 100 less calories for their kids compared with families who didn't have nutritional information (calorie count) on the menu. Just by having the number of calories listed for each food item on the menu, families made better choices for their child.

Brilliant and then seemingly simple. However, lots of fast-food chains still don't readily provide nutritional information. As menu-labeling laws may be incorporated into health care change and reform, this study helps define how important access to nutritional information is for all of us.

One-hundred calories may not seem like a big deal. It is. Over time, just eating an excess of 100 calories every day can cause a child to get fat.

One-hundred extra calories a day can mean everything when you're weighing in at around 30 to 40 pounds in the preschooler ring.

One way I like to think about overeating is the concept of *energy gap*. Energy gap represents the imbalance of energy (food) taken in and energy that is expended (calories burned off). Kids get overweight because they eat more food and calories (energy in) than the calories they need to grow, develop, and function on a daily basis (energy out). This excess energy intake is an abundance or gap in energy balance.

The goal is, of course, for all of us to have our

ENERGY IN = ENERGY OUT
(food + drinks)   **(growth + energy to play and move + daily functioning)**

For healthy, growing children, finding equivalence in this equation can be a huge challenge in the face of large portion sizes, snacks galore (more energy in), and more time in front of the computer and TV (less expenditure).

Data on energy gap are kind of astounding to parents when I share them.

For example, it's not often the case that an overweight 3-year-old is pigging out all day and lying around watching TV. More, it seems, for overweight children and teens, weight gain may be much more insidious that that. Overweight tends to sneak up on kids and families when they don't even know it's happening! Often parents can't believe their child is in the overweight or unhealthy weight category when I tell them. Thinking about trimming off 100 calories here or there may be the difference in keeping a family healthy over time.

Energy gap research finds that for kids between ages 2 and 7 years, it only takes an excess of about 110 to 165 calories a day to make them fat over time! Abnormal weight gain is often accumulated over time and occurs over days and days. Using the assumption that 3,500 extra calories leads to an average of 1-lb weight gain as fat, researchers found that a reduction in the energy gap of 110 to 165 calories/day could have prevented kids between the ages of 2 and 7 years from gaining excess weight and putting them at risk for being overweight.

Yowsers. That 100 calories you save your child while watching portions and making good choices while keeping calorie counts in mind in the grocery store or at home (or even when at McDonald's) will really make a difference over time.

Another fine example that our instincts can serve us well. *When we have the right information (say, calorie count and food labels that tell us what we are eating), we can do a good job making better choices for our kids.*

That 100 calories a day may really subtract down into an equality of energy intake and expenditure, leading to overall improved health for years to come.

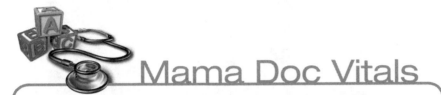

Mama Doc Vitals

Study: Energy gap data from study in *Pediatrics* (http://bit.ly/mdm-EnergyGap): "Consistent behavioral changes averaging 110 to 165 kcal/day may be sufficient to counterbalance the energy gap. Changes in excess dietary intake (eg, eliminating one sugar-sweetened beverage at 150 kcal per can) may be easier to attain than increases in physical activity levels (eg, a 30-kg boy replacing sitting for 1.9 hours with 1.9 hours walking for an extra 150 kcal)."

Fact: An Oreo cookie has 80 calories per cookie. Just 2 less Oreos a day and you may decrease the energy gap!

Tip: Involve your children in reading labels—my boys love to compare the sugar content in cereals, for example! Take the time to look at the calorie and nutrition information on packages, wrappers, and menus when available, especially if you and your child ever find yourselves under the glow of the golden arches—those 100 calories mean something.

7

Why Broad-spectrum Sunscreen?

More important than any granular, scientific detail about a sunscreen ingredient, UV-A/UV-B radiation, or its vehicle—if the sunscreen comes as a spray, a lotion, or an ointment—is how you use it. *The best sunscreen is the one that is used early and often on children.* No sunscreen is waterproof, and no sunscreen is play proof. For infants and toddlers, I've found the best trick for easy application is to put it on while they are strapped into the car seat on your way to the beach! There's no controversy that it's best to apply sunscreen 20 minutes before sun exposure and repeat the application head to toe every 2 hours during active play/swim. (See Chapter 8 for information on babies younger than 6 months.)

> Don't forget that sun-protective clothing decreases the amount of sunscreen you'll have to use. Start putting your baby in long-sleeved ultraviolet (UV)-protective clothing from day one of swimming. You'll then not need to use as much sunscreen because much of your baby's body will be covered.

Also, don't be fooled—sunscreens marketed for children may not provide any increased safety or protection. You'll see and hear conflicting reports on ingredient safety, particularly as differing groups discuss concerns about chemical ingredients versus physical/mineral ingredients. Trouble is, groups now warn about the physical/mineral ingredients (previously felt to be the safest) due to their particle size. And although the US Food and Drug Administration (FDA) warns against using spray sunscreen with children (concerns about inhalation of the fumes), most families love the convenience. So if you love the spray, have your children hold their breath while you apply it.

> *The best sunscreen is the one that is used early and often on children.*

Good thing is, most everyone agrees that the ingredients in sunscreen are less risky than any significant sun exposure or burn in childhood.

Eight Tips for Buying and Using Sunscreen on Children

1. It's not the brand or the sun protection factor (SPF) number that matters the most. What matters most is how you use sunscreen. Apply sunscreen about a half hour before your kids go outside. It is absorbed into the skin better this way.

2. You'll need to look for a sunscreen that has 2 or 3 ingredients to cover all the range of UV-A and UV-B rays that damage our skin.

3. Fortunately, in 2013 the FDA changed regulations so sunscreen manufacturers can't make false claims. That being said, don't trust the "sweatproof, waterproof" claims. Reapply sunscreen every 2 hours if your kids are playing actively, swimming, and sweating. When you reapply, pay attention to areas that burn a lot—shoulders, back, chest, ears, nose, and lips.

4. Those sunscreens marketed for kids may not be any safer than adult brands. "Tear-free" may not be tear-free either unless no chemical ingredients are used. So use caution around your baby's or toddler's eyes. Using a hat will help as there're less need for perfect application around the eyes if you're in the shade!

5. Be an ingredient hound. Look for sunscreen with SPF 30 to 50 that covers full UV-A and UV-B. If you're worried about chemical exposure, look for those that use zinc or titanium as the barrier for sunscreen. Those metals or physical barriers are not absorbed into your child's skin.

6. Don't be stingy; use a lot of sunscreen—a shot-glass size for a body, even a little body like your child.

7. Avoid the most direct and dangerous midday sun whenever you can. Keep kids out of the sun between 10:00 am and 3:00 to 4:00 pm. I know, this sounds crazy, as children love to play outdoors midday. You can follow the UV index online or via SunWise apps. These apps tell you the hourly UV index during the day for your zip code—amazingly informative.

8. If you can, get a UV swimsuit, a hat, and sunglasses to protect your kids. If it's the norm and you start them early, the battles will be small. Kids will never think it's funny to have a hat on in the sun if they have always done it that way.

Loving the sun is not the problem. It's sensible to crave sunlight; the sun promotes feelings of well-being, while sunlight is essential for vitamin D synthesis in our skin, which can mediate mood among all sorts of other goodness.

The sun provides UV radiation, however, so we need to balance the benefits of sunlight with the risks of UV radiation, particularly in children. Ultraviolet radiation is harmful because it damages skin, and evidence supports a strong causal relationship between sunlight exposure and skin cancer. In particular, there is a heightened risk of melanoma for those with increased childhood sun exposure. Ultraviolet radiation is made up of UV-A and UV-B waves of light. *This is handy:* UV-B light is the light that **B**urns, and UV-A light is the light that causes your skin to **A**ge (wrinkle).

WendySueSwanson MD @SeattleMamaDoc

Will do everything I can to prevent my boys fr having the melanoma I had. 1 severe sunburn as kid 2X risk of melanoma

---

A Little Science About UV-A/UV-B Light and Sunscreen

- UV-A radiation causes **A**ging and deeper skin damage. To protect against the entire spectrum of UV-A rays, you'll likely need 2 ingredients in the sunscreen—most commonly you will see oxybenzone or avobenzone coupled with another (eg, zinc oxide, titanium dioxide) to cover the entire UV-A spectrum of light. Although some people report concerns about oxybenzone irritation to sensitive skin, recent research finds that when it's only at the typical 1% to 6% concentrations, skin reactions are unlikely. If using a sunscreen for the first time, apply a small patch of sunscreen to your child's leg as a test before using it elsewhere. UV-A radiation is constant throughout the year, regardless of season or heat index.

- UV-B radiation causes **B**urning. The SPF you see on sunscreen bottles and clothing relates to the ability of the sunscreen to protect you from UV-B light. Pick anything with an SPF over 30 as it protects against about 97% of the UV-B light. You can get 60 to 90 SPF, but most experts agree you aren't getting much more bang for your buck. UV-B radiation varies with the season (unlike UV-A)—it's most intense in the summer.

If you hate the idea of chemicals or even metals on your children's skin, consider using other barriers to reduce the amount of sunscreen you're forced to use.

Ways to Reduce Sunscreen Use While Still Providing Protection

1. Cover your children up with hats and long sleeves whenever you can to reduce the amount of skin you need to cover with sunscreen. Do the same for yourself. It's remarkably easier to get the boys to wear a hat when I do too.

2. Stay out of the sun (when you can) between 10:00 am and 4:00 pm as the sun is most intense and UV radiation is highest during peak hours. Follow the UV index.

3. Take a bath before bed on the days you apply sunscreen—get rid of all those physical and chemical ingredients from the skin when you're done using them!

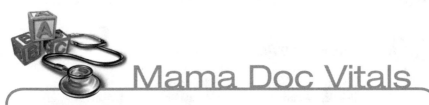

Mama Doc Vitals

Power Parent: Make it a new habit to follow the UV index daily. Check it like you check the weather. Know the strength of the sun: http://bit.ly/mdm-sunwise.

Tip: Use hats and UV-protective clothing for the majority of your infant's or child's body. That'll leave less fighting for the face and other body parts you'll need to cover with sunscreen.

Fact: One severe sunburn during childhood doubles your child's risk of malignant melanoma.

8

Protecting Babies From the Sun

Here's why to avoid sunscreen for babies younger than 6 months (when you can) and ways to protect babies from the sun...

We know that early exposure to excessive sun in infants and toddlers increases their likelihood of malignant cancer later in life. We also know that all types of skin cancer are increased in the United States. There was a great new insight paper that came out in June 2011 that helped me understand the whys behind the recommendation for no sunscreen before 6 months. Here's what we know. Infant skin versus adult skin is really different. It's thinner, it lacks as many melanocytes, or those cells that put melanin or pigment in your skin. Because of that, it's more vulnerable to the penetrating UV light that comes and hits our skin. It's also more vulnerable for absorbing the chemicals that are in sunscreens. The less sun coupled with the least chemicals is ideal.

Whenever possible, cover babies younger than 6 months with hats, long sleeves, visors that are on strollers, and umbrellas. Enjoy the planet with your baby but know there's no benefit for direct sun. If you get yourself in a position where you're going to be out in the direct sunshine and you don't think every part of your baby will be protected, that's when you should use sunscreen. Sunscreen prior to 6 months is typically unnecessary. However, if your infant is going to have direct sun exposure, test a physical blocker sunscreen on her arm or leg. You should always use a sunscreen of SPF greater than 30. It doesn't have to be marketed toward children, but you might want "tear-free" if you're going to use it on the face.

Only apply it to the areas that will be exposed outside of the sleeves and hat that you have on. Cover exposed areas well but certainly not skin under sun-protective clothing. Because we know the effects of that sunscreen and the chemicals that are in them may be more readily absorbed, use it only when you have to on an infant!

Mama Doc Vitals

Tip: For more information about using sunscreen in infants and older children, check out "Sun Safety" at HealthyChildren.org for ingredient information, tips for getting sunscreen on, and an explanation about UV-A/UV-B: http://bit.ly/mdm-SunSafety.

Tip: Don't forget about the power of shade! Before infants crawl, it's typically easy to contain them under the shade of an umbrella, stroller, or sun-protective clothing.

9

If It Were My Child:
No Television in the Bedroom

While I was getting ready for the day when Oden was 2½ years old, I let him watch *Sesame Street*. In the show, the segments change every few minutes or so and seem to weave old-school 1970s content (familiar to me) with newly created vignettes that have a modern feel and construction. I liked it nearly as much as the boys. One of the stories we saw was about tooth fairies. An animated group of fairies (Abby's Fairy Flying School) were detailing how they got to the tooth under a child's pillow (lifting up the child) to replace it with a golden coin. Mind you, I was coming and going from the room and didn't view the whole story. However, at one point, the fairies accidentally turn on the child's TV and worry it might wake the child, ultimately uncovering their work and secret magic.

A TV in the child's bedroom? No way, Sesame.

If it were my child, I'd never allow a TV in the child's bedroom. Plain and simple, I know it's not good for children and ultimately will only detract from their life. When I talk to families in clinic, I say that TV in the bedroom is just never going to make their life *better*. It won't really enhance. Unfortunately, what I hear is that it might make a parent's life better. Some families really do come to rely on it, as did I this morning while I was getting ready. But we need to figure out ways to use it better. When I talk with families about reducing media time, I talk about media use and the substantial effect junk-food advertising has on children actually asking for and eating junk food, how distracted eating (eating in front of a screen) may contribute to obesity, how TV contributes to disrupted and poor quality of sleep, and studies that find early TV exposure increases the risk of attention challenges. TV on in the background or on while a child is playing doesn't help language development either.

TV can be a great way for children to learn cooperation and model friendship or empathy if shown educational programming geared for their age. In balance, TV isn't all bad, and some research shows "pro-social" content can help children learn to trust adults and improve their behavior scores. Of course we make screen time decisions in the context of life.

But I must say, I really don't think TV will make your child smarter.

The timing of this Sesame episode I mentioned was uncanny. The very same day, the American Academy of Pediatrics published a policy statement from the Council on Communications and Media (full disclosure: I sit on this council) entitled, "Children, Adolescents, Obesity, and the Media," detailing effects of screen time/media and junk-food advertising on children in relation to obesity. The authors state, "Sufficient evidence exists to warrant a ban on junk-food or fast-food advertising in children's TV programming," and they point out, "Pediatricians need to ask 2 questions about media use at every well-child or well-adolescent visit: (1) How much screen time is being spent per day? and (2) Is there a TV set or Internet connection in the child's bedroom?"

> **I really don't think TV will make your child smarter.**

I also tell families that TV watching is not as cognitively sedating as our instincts may suggest. TV viewing in the 1 to 2 hours before bed seems to rev kids up, not wind them down. There's even more data to support this. Michelle Garrison, PhD; Kimberly Liekweg, BA; and Dimitri Christakis, MD, MPH, FAAP, published a study in *Pediatrics* describing violent TV's effect on preschoolers. They studied more than 600 children between 3 and 5 years of age and reviewed their TV/media diaries.

- Garrison et al found that preschoolers watched on average more than an hour of TV daily (72.9 minutes), with the minority being at bedtime (14 minutes after 7:00 pm).
- They also found that children with a bedroom TV watched 40 more minutes of TV than those without one. Not surprisingly, children with a bedroom TV watched more TV after 7:00 pm as well.
- Violent TV viewing in the daytime and TV after 7:00 pm disrupted sleep for the preschoolers.
- Children with a bedroom TV were more likely to have parent-reported daytime tiredness (8% versus 1% without bedroom TV).
- Children were more likely to have trouble falling asleep, more nightmares, and more awakenings if in the hour prior to going to bed, they watched TV, violent or not.

- Fortunately, nonviolent daytime TV didn't seem to change or impair preschoolers' sleep.
- It didn't make a difference on sleep if parents watched TV alongside their children.

WendySueSwanson MD @SeattleMamaDoc

In clinic, I ask teens if they sleep with their cell phones.

A TV (or iPad, computer, or smartphone) in the bedroom makes pre-bedtime viewing that much more common. Once a screen is in a child's room, it will be difficult to get it out. Most estimates find that about a third of every preschooler in America has a TV in the bedroom (some studies as high as 40%). So something about this is very appealing to many families. A really tough habit to break.

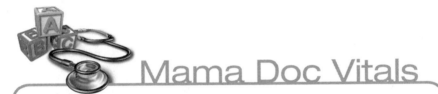

Mama Doc Vitals

Tip: No screens 2 hours before bed. The light from the screen tends to decrease melatonin release in the brain—that hormone that helps our brains chill out for the night.

Fact: Children younger than 11 years spend more than 3 hours with screens every day in the United States. About one-third of toddlers in the United States have a TV in their bedroom.

Tip: A screen that plays videos (such as a tablet, iPad, or smartphone) should be considered a TV and shouldn't sleep in the bedroom.

10

What Does Television Do to My Kid's Brain?

If you want to understand more about the effects of TV on the brain, you need to watch a talk by Dimitri Christakis, MD, MPH, FAAP, who is a pediatric researcher. The science around TV viewing and its effect on children and concentration astound me. Not because any of it is counterintuitive, but because TV is as powerful as it is. Television is a large part of most children's lives here in the United States, and this presentation of fact and observations may change what you do at home.

Although it seems like there is no controversy here, I've stumbled on more than one mom proclaiming the benefits for TV at bedtime from infancy up online. People love the convenience of TV. And infants, toddlers, and school-aged children are of course drawn into watching the images when they come up.

We gotta get the word out on the science.

A Few Takeaways on Media and Early Learning

- Early experiences condition the mind. Connections between brain cells change based on experiences our children have while their brain triples in size between birth and age 3.
- Initiation of television viewing is now (on average) 4 months of age.
- Prolonged exposure to rapid image changes (like on a TV show designed for an infant) during critical periods of brain development may precondition the mind to expect high levels of stimulation. This may then make the pace of *real life* less able to sustain our children's attention. The more hours a child views rapid-fire television, the more likely he will have attention challenges later in life.
- Cognitive stimulation (reading books or going to a museum) reduces the likelihood of attention challenges later in life.
- What content your child watches on TV matters—the more frenetic or violent the TV show, the more likely your child will have attention challenges later in life. Television shows that move at a typical pace may be far better for our children.

- New studies (using mice) may demonstrate that learning suffers with excess TV viewing.
- We need more real-time play for children. (Get out the blocks or get outside!)

I'd suggest the 15 minutes or so it takes to view the talk might profoundly change your thinking about TV. Many parents in clinic who have watched the video have told me this. Direct from the mouth of a father, pediatrician, and researcher, Dr Christakis explains how the brain develops and what TV may do and theorizes why ample time in front of the TV as an infant or toddler may reorganize how a child thinks and solves problems. More than anything, watching this made me want to reverse time and go back to do even more for my little boys and their developing brains. If only the daily museum trip was plausible…

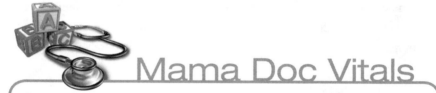

Mama Doc Vitals

Watch: Dr Christakis' amazing talk about TV and children's brain development: http://bit.ly/mdm-TVbrain

Tip: Television in the background matters too. If the TV is on while a child is playing, she tends to look up and get distracted, thus interfering with thinking and focus.

11

What Your Child Watches on Television Matters

A 2011 *Pediatrics* study about the effects of watching fast-paced cartoons on the attention and working memory of 4-year-olds caught my attention. It's basically a SpongeBob versus Crayola versus Caillou showdown. At least it feels that way to me. And thus, it's bound to hit the front pages of every parent's windshield at one point or another. First and foremost, it was a genius study for getting the word out and attracting media attention—media love to talk about media. Especially when it comes to the effects on children; all forms of media are looking for a viable option for longevity. There is just so much competition now.

We watched *Caillou* in our house for a while and my husband and I liked to dissect and ridicule it after the boys were in bed. It's frumpy and moves so flipping slow—everything from the outfits to the color scheme to the lessons. As a parent, it's painful to watch—it's just so utterly wholesome. On the flip side, because of this goodness in the content and pace, we feel less "guilty" letting the boys watch it. The result has been a win-win: the boys used to looooooove it—I mean, love it—and we would pat ourselves on the back for the choice.

Good media is far better than bad media. If moderation is king, guilt-free is queen.

Fortunately, data back up our instinct. And this helps with our mommy-daddy guilt. We're a really low media-viewing house but not the lowest. We have friends whose children don't see a screen for months at a time.

The findings are not at all surprising. If you sat down a group of parents in a room and asked which they thought was better for their child's memory, attention, and performance on tasks—A) coloring; B) watching *Caillou*; or C) watching *SpongeBob SquarePants*—I suspect they would all come up with the results in the study. However, the beauty of the research is that it puts us one step closer in understanding why fast-paced shows may render our children less attentive, less focused, and impatient in the real world.

The study provides data, confirms instinct, and fuels efforts for me at home and in clinic. It serves up ammo for my "Think about *what* your kids are watching in addition to how much they are watching" advice for parents. I think you'll find the study design fascinating too. The details matter here.

Because the results aren't surprising (watching fast-paced cartoons hindered attention, focus, and memory), it's more helpful to look at the methods and data and see what it means for you and your family individually.

Researchers in Virginia took a group of sixty 4-year-olds and randomly assigned them to 1 of 3 groups. Children were then put in a room alone and asked to draw with crayons, watch *Caillou* (a PBS show), or watch *SpongeBob SquarePants* (a Nickelodeon show) for 9 minutes on a computer.

> For fun, search Caillou and SpongeBob on the Internet to see how different these shows are represented online. The online user experience for these shows couldn't be more different.

Immediately after the 9-minute intervention, children completed a battery of tests that required focus, concentration, patience, a working memory, and manipulation. Researchers asked children to rearrange blocks with certain rules; they were asked to follow complicated commands like, "When I say touch your head, I want you to touch your toes, but when I say touch your toes, I want you to touch your head"; and participate in the marshmallow test, a delayed-gratification task. The marshmallow test is the most intoxicating to think about. Basically, children are left in a room with a bowl of marshmallows or Goldfish crackers to decide which they like. On one plate are 10 marshmallows; on the other plate are only 2. Children are told that if they wait until the experimenter returns, they get to eat all 10. If they ring a bell early, the experimenter will come back into the room right away, but they will only get to eat the plate with 2. In the past, the marshmallow test has been used to predict school performance and has even been found to predict performance on the SAT some 18 years later. Watch an example of the marshmallow test. It's a delightful test to observe.

The Results

Groups didn't differ in attention skills/problems at the outset based on parent reports prior to the study. Because kids were randomly assigned to each group, the groups were thought to be very alike.

Children who watched the fast-paced TV did significantly worse on the attention and memory testing. There was no difference in performance between the educational TV *(Caillou)* group versus the drawing group.

Delay of gratification (the marshmallow test) was analyzed separately and measured in the number of seconds waited before eating the marshmallow. The children who watched *SpongeBob SquarePants* did significantly worse than the drawing and *Caillou*-watching groups. Again, the *Caillou* group performed equally to the drawing group.

Researchers don't know exactly why the SpongeBob watchers did so poorly. They theorize it has to do with rapid-fire motion, the only seconds-long scenes, and the fact that kids don't have to really engage in the content. Although somewhat controversial, there have been many studies finding that fast-paced media at a young age may lead to inattention later in life. So working off of that, researchers theorize that SpongeBob is superfast moving and unlike any cogent interaction or experience in the real world.

The limitations?

It was a very small study. Only 60 children participated. Further, the kids were all white and from upper-middle- and middle-class families. Although this may project well on decisions in my home, it may not for my friends with different backgrounds or many of my patients. Further, the group of kids in the study had parents who had time to do this—which already puts them in a curious group!

The children watched for only 9 minutes of the show. We don't know what happens to their working memory, concentration level, and attention if they watch the whole 30-minute show or hours of similar shows. Further, the testing was done immediately after watching, and so we don't know what happens to their brain as time unfolds. Is the effect transient?

Nickelodeon states that SpongeBob isn't designed for 4-year-olds even though we know young children (even younger than 4) tend to love it! Further research on older children may help us understand if the disruption in executive function happens in a critical time of development (eg, younger than age 6) or if fast-paced cartoon viewing is detrimental to school performance, memory, and attention all the way through childhood.

What to Do: Cartoons on the Brain

This really isn't about one show over another. This isn't about trashing one cartoon network either. It's about harnessing information that helps us make media-savvy decisions for our children and helps us raise media-savvy adults who know how to thrive online and offline. We weren't reared on SpongeBob and iPads, smartphones and Nintendo DS, or DVDs and the Wii. Yes, we had TV, but we consumed about half the hours children today consume. So our job today is to guide our children into a place of balance with media. Media (in its beauty and its beast) is here to stay. In many regards, children will need to function at a fast-paced, digital-literate pace to be successful as they grow up and transition to adults. So what we model, what we choose to expose our children to, and how much we let them sit in front of screens is relevant. Learning to find balance and compartmentalize our media is key. This isn't a keep-away-from-technology book chapter.

But…

We want our children to have intimate, authentic, personal friendships. We want them to know how to learn online but also offline, in the silences of the woods and a silent well-run classroom. We want them to look their friends and partners in the eyes. We want them to experience the beautiful part of an uninterrupted conversation.

My advice?

- If it were my child, I'd observe how your children behave, listen, function, and learn after watching TV.
- With the data from this study, I wouldn't let them watch fast-paced cartoons just before school, just before sitting down to dinner with your family, or just before bed.
- I'd rip out excess TVs in your home. I'd never put one in a child's bedroom. I'd limit screen time to about an hour a day throughout all of childhood.
- I'd choose naturally paced shows for preschoolers that hold educational value like *Sesame Street* or a favorite in our home, *Driver Dan's Story Train*.
- You know all this already. If your kids have watched 230 hours of SpongeBob? They'll be fine. Your children won't grow up to be unemployed, inattentive, inconsiderate humans by watching one particular cartoon. However, I believe they may be more balanced, more focused, and better students and friends if you limit their exposure to this fast-paced media from here forward.

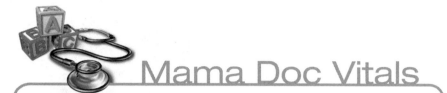

Mama Doc Vitals

Watch: The marshmallow test—it's a delightful test to observe: http://bit.ly/mdm-MarshmallowTest.

Tip: Good media use is a blend of good content and moderation. Stop feeling guilty. If moderation is king, guilt-free is queen! Find a balance for your family and do your best to stick to it.

12

Why No Television Before Bed Is Better

Television before bed delays children going to sleep. We've all heard that TV isn't necessarily good for our children right before bed, but something about that fact tends to go against instinct. In my experience, most of us feel like TV and video streaming are relaxing to our minds. Bum news is, it's the opposite. Viewing TV or video or screens prior to sleep tends to rev up our brains and disrupt our sleep and may even cause nightmares (especially for preschoolers). The light from computers and screens may inhibit melatonin, the hormone that helps us drift off to sleep. A 2013 *Pediatrics* study reminds us about TV realities at bedtime.

I'm as guilty as everyone else. I love to let my children watch a TV show after dinner in the hour before bed. We all crave that downtime with our full bellies and the work of our day behind us. We all want some quiet. But here's the thing…

Researchers surveyed more than 2,000 children between 5 and 24 years of age. They inquired about the last 1½ hours of their day—not surprisingly, they found that TV before bed was common. Across all ages, watching TV was the most common activity for children before bed, and about half of the children watched TV for at least 30 minutes. When they surveyed what time children went to sleep, they confirmed the concerns about TV and bedtime. The children with more TV viewing went to sleep later. Conversely, those with an earlier bedtime had significantly greater time in non-screen sedentary activities and self-care prior to going to sleep. Most research shows that our children's sleep deprivation is due to late bedtimes, not early rising. Children sleep about 1 hour less now than they did 100 years ago. Consequently, we're also more fatigued, distracted, obese, and hyperactive these days—all things associated with sleep loss. Strategies that help us go to sleep on time are essential for our very tired country.

Television Tips to Improve Our Children's Sleep

- If your child is having trouble falling asleep, work hard to make sure she doesn't spend any time in front of a screen 2 hours prior to bedtime. Explain to her why you're doing this—the TV winds them up, not down.
- Get all screens out of the room where your children sleep. No TVs, cell phones, tablets, or iPods in bedrooms or in bed with children. Make rules for a sleeping station for phones in your kitchen. Phones go to bed at, say, 9:00 pm.
- Buy a new alarm clock if a child says that the phone must wake her up in the morning. I find alarm clocks online for less than $15.
- If your child loves TV, shift the time of day she watches TV. Consider using all screens as devices of privilege. Let children earn an hour with their TV or video game while you prepare dinner for great citizenship at home or school.

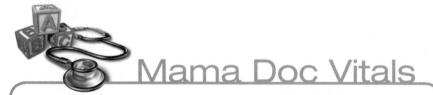

Mama Doc Vitals

Study: Preschool activities and timing of sleep: http://bit.ly/mdm-presleep

Tip: Remind caregivers, babysitters, and grandparents that screens impair melatonin release. Screens before bed make it harder for children to fall asleep.

Parent Power: Don't let children and teens convince you they need their smartphone in the bedroom because of the clock.

13

Asking About Guns in Your House

Asking friends about guns is a little like asking about their underwear. Not in the pediatric office, but at home, on the street, and in the neighborhood.

My old next-door neighbor (NDN) is a stay-at-home dad (SAHD). On most days, he runs his household and wrangles 8- and 6-year-old boys until his wife joins him after work. The 3 (or 4) of them seem to weave and pedal through life, on and off their bikes. I can see them coming and going throughout the day; it's my crystal ball of sorts as to what life with 2 boys may look like about 5 years from now.

> *It's always what we don't think of that takes our breath away while raising kids.*

My NDN once approached me from his porch. When we lived on the same street we'd often talk, porch to porch, about life, the trees, our favorite noodle shop, or the weather. He said, "You should write a post about gun violence." I said, "Yeah, I know, I should write about 2 million posts about gun violence." This was 2010 and well before the Newtown, CT, shootings and the time in which I feel the national dialogue really seemed to change here in the United States.

But then he framed the issue for me. And I knew he was right—I had to write about it.

His 8-year-old had just come home from a friend's house. While playing at the boy's home, the two 8-year-olds came upon a BB gun. They thought it was loaded. Knowing exactly what it was, NDN's son convinced his friend not to touch it (or so the story goes). He came home and told his dad the saga. NDN was stunned. It's always what we don't think of that takes our breath away while raising kids. NDN never thought he left his child in a dangerous situation when he dropped him off to play. Hearing about the BB gun made him wonder if he should be asking more questions.

As I got to thinking about it, I went back out to the porch. We talked about it a bit more. At the time my kids were young; we weren't yet dropping them off for playdates. But suddenly I instantly knew the dilemma. First on the list of questions for a generous family that would invite my child into its home for an afternoon wouldn't be, "Do you have a gun in the house?" It's a seemingly personal question for some reason. Almost like, "Does your wife wear lacy underwear?"

Point is, it feels like a personal question. But it's also a practical one. And it may be a necessary one too. More than 8 million children have access to firearms in our country. The American Academy of Pediatrics says, "Even if you don't have guns in your own home, that won't eliminate your child's risks. Half of the homes in the United States contain firearms, and more than a third of all accidental shootings of children take place in the homes of their friends, neighbors, or relatives."

NDN's story about the BB gun helped drive the point home for me.

Of course, we do all sorts of uncomfortable things to protect our children. It starts with pregnancy, followed closely by losing all sense of a personal life while raising toddlers, and rounds off with paying for college and perhaps a wedding. But asking about guns in the homes of their friends is one of those things I've never thought to talk about in clinic.

Protecting Your Children From Firearms

- Get over it being awkward to ask about guns. Asking about guns saves lives. It isn't underwear. Ask supervising parents if they have guns in their home before playdates or sleepovers. Don't make assumptions; ask relatives too.
- It's my belief that guns have no place in a home with children. I remember the 16-year-old sibling of a classmate who shot himself. I remember my middle school student who was shot and killed just outside the middle school I taught at in 1997. Before you hold up your National Rifle Association signs or start your internal rant, I'll say this: if there is a gun in a home and I'm (or you're) not going to change that, there are things you can do to protect yourself, your children, and your community.
- If a gun is in your home, it should be stored unloaded, in a locked case, and inaccessible to children. Ammunition should be stored separately. Hide the keys to the case.

- BB guns are guns. And if your child has access to the Internet, they can make one. I searched for "BB gun" on Google and found all sorts of information, including links on how to make your own gun. The reality is that it is your job to talk with children about guns—early and often.

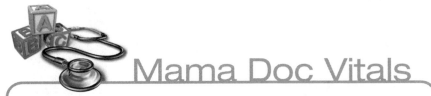

Mama Doc Vitals

Link: "Handguns in the Home": http://bit.ly/mdm-GunSafety

Tip: Always ask about guns before a playdate or sleepover. From experience I'll tell you that it gets easier and easier to ask. Not all parents will experience the question as threatening or judgmental.

Fact: A home without guns is a safer home. But truth is, 40% of homes with children in the United States have guns in them. We all have to help keep them out of kids' reach.

14

About Violent Video Games

"We don't benefit from ignorance. We don't benefit from not knowing the science of this epidemic of violence," President Obama said in 2013 after the Newtown, CT, shootings. "…Congress should fund research into the effects that violent video games have on young minds."

Only a month after the Newtown tragedy, I was pleased to hear the President's plan to decrease gun violence and his steadfast effort to improve the safety of our communities by decreasing violence, death, and suffering from firearms. Delighted to hear that the government is looking to ensure that it's safe to talk about firearm safety in the examination room (at a federal level) and also that he's implored Congress to study the effects of video games on young minds. That being said, we do know a bit about the effects of video games on young minds. An American Academy of Pediatrics 2009 "Media Violence" policy statement noted,

"The strength of the association between media violence and aggressive behavior found on meta-analyses is greater than the association between calcium intake and bone mass, lead ingestion and lower IQ, and condom nonuse and sexually acquired HIV infection, and is nearly as strong as the association between cigarette smoking and lung cancer—associations that clinicians accept and on which preventive medicine is based without question."

To be clear, the $10 million that President Obama granted (at press time, closer to $130 million, pending senate approval) the Centers for Disease Control and Prevention to investigate the effects of violent video games on our children is not a ton of money. And the tone, according to Stephen Dinan of *The Washington Times,* places more responsibility in our hands—"…overall, the White House said that while limiting guns is the role of the government, controlling what Americans see in movies and games is best left to parents."

As parents and pediatricians, community members and mentors, and American citizens, there are things we can do now to improve our children's exposure to and absorption of violence.

Thoughts on Children's Massive Exposure to Violence

- Data find that witnessing violent acts in the media (in a game, TV, or video) can contribute to aggressive behavior, desensitization to violence, nightmares, and fear of being harmed. Research finds, "Consistent and significant associations between media exposure and increases in aggression and violence have been found in American and cross-cultural studies; in field experiments, laboratory experiments, cross-sectional studies, and longitudinal studies; and with children, adolescents, and young adults."

- We need to know more about what video games do to our brains. That being said, when video games reward killing of humans in more and more realistic ways, they may teach children to associate pleasure with the suffering or killing of others. This just can't be a good way to spend hours a day as a developing human. More research will help us understand this better, yet previous research has found that first-person–shooting experiences desensitize and divorce us from the act of killing.

- Ages matters. Children 8 years and younger have a difficult time sorting out fantasy from fiction. Don't allow young children access to or let them witness violent games that involve shooting and killing. During the same week as President Obama's proclamation, an online app branded with the National Rifle Association name was released online advertised for children 4 years and up. Due to public outcry, 2 days after the app launch, developers changed the recommended age to 12 years and older. My opinion: game makers may not be looking out for your child.

- We need to consider following the rating of video games more aggressively. Parents can insist a child is 17 years old to play a 17-and-up game.

- Children 8 to 18 spend more than 6 hours a day using entertainment media (TV, computer, video, movies, radio, music). Consider limiting children's time with screens to the recommended 2 hours or less. If that's exceedingly difficult, take baby steps. Step one: consider limiting time with violent video games today. Get them out of the house—don't allow teens to play them online. The majority of fourth- to 12th-grade students report playing games with an ESRB rating of M for Mature (recommended only for those older than 17). Further, 78% of boys younger than 17 report owning M-rated games.

- By 18, an average child has seen 200,000 acts of violence on TV alone. Watch TV with your children when you can and turn it off when it gets gnarly.

- Exposure to violent media can have lasting effects. Exposure to violence can potentially lead to anxiety, depression, post-traumatic stress disorder, sleep trouble, and nightmares. Work to turn off the TV 2 hours before bed to help children sleep. If they have nightmares, are anxious or depressed, or are suffering from signs of increasing stress, talk with their doctor. Talk with your children and teens about creating a "media diet"—a fair way for them to watch media in a balanced way. You can help restrict violent media. Your children really do care what you think.

What Parents Need to Know

- Violent video games may change your child's perception of aggression and may desensitize him or her to violent acts.
- Play games before your children buy or download them. Know what your children play online and at home, then let them know your reflections.
- Observe and follow video game ratings. Use Common Sense Media as a resource for looking up and reviewing video, movies, and games. Common Sense Media has an app I like too.
- Set limits. Especially for online gaming.
- Have kids play video games together, not alone.
- Think about a healthy media diet. Strive to reduce media after dinner (in the 2 hours before bed) and work to help your children find a bit of balance with video games, TV viewing, movies, and online videos.

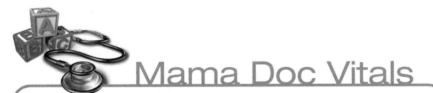

Mama Doc Vitals

Tip: There are data that find that children and teens can be desensitized to violence on TV and in video games, apps, or online sites. Play with your child and make rules together about what is acceptable at home.

Fact: Children 8 to 18 years of age spend 6 hours with entertainment media every day. This is a big part of their lives. Shaping rules and providing insight for your kids is a good use of your time.

App/Link: Use Common Sense Media to read about, rate, and make decisions about video games (www.commonsensemedia.org).

Link: Check out Entertainment Software Rating Board ratings, now required for all video games, at www.esrb.org.

15

Going Back to School Monday After Newtown Shootings

As the Monday after the Newtown shootings approached and we readied our children for school, most of us had a little bit of dread in our hearts. I did. There was unease as we returned our children to school.

The few days around the time of the shootings were bewildering. Making sense of the tragedy in Connecticut was a huge challenge, particularly as the details of the shooting simultaneously unfolded alongside the details of the beautiful lost children and educators. There's little more to say than it was tragic and head-shaking. There is just no sense to what unfolded here in America. And although there are stories of incredible heroism, we are left mourning and aching. Still.

In my 4+ years using social media at that point, no single topic had ever overrun my channels like the shooting. We were all aghast and terrified, sad and stunned. As President Obama said, "We're heartbroken." When I opened the Sunday *New York Times* after the shooting, I gulped and teared up again— I simply couldn't wrap my head around the number of 6- and 7-year-olds we'd lost. Especially as one sat next to me at the breakfast table.

The randomness of this event allowed us all to relate to the details of the horror and loss with uncomfortable familiarity.

We can and will work toward a safer future for our children. Don't ease up on yourself or those in your community for action—improved communication, access to mental health, examining gun control—as months unfold. The future keeps coming quickly.

Tips for Children Going Back to School After Tragedies

- **Your child's school is safe.** The fact remains that a horrific shooting or tragedy is an anomaly. Your child's school is a very safe place to be. Remind yourself, and your children if they ask, that a tragedy is typically an exception.
- **Get the information you need to feel safe.** Send an e-mail to the principal, your children's teacher, or fellow parents—perhaps commit to participating in ensuring you have good safety measures in place at your school. Leaving

a voice message, sending an e-mail, or joining the community of families wanting to ensure safety as the days unfold will likely ease your fears. Get involved. Write a letter to the President (The White House, 1600 Pennsylvania Ave NW, Washington, DC 20500) or your congressional representative. Action after tragedy is an antidote to anxiety.

- **Take breaks from media reports.** Like any overwhelming informational stream, we need to compartmentalize. Our curiosity for details is human. This stems from our compassion for our own children. Yet relentless consumption will only steep anxiety and heartache.

- **Sketch out a plan for today right now.** Think about your ideal day. When do you want to hear news updates, or not? If information and news updates about a specific tragedy help you feel secure, incorporate updates into your day. But space them out so that you have blocks of time with no information flow. Close the Facebook window at work; watch the news only for a half hour at a time. Your own stress to any tragedy is very important for your children too. Check in with your school in the morning and with media at a time when you can deal with it. Otherwise, return to your daily routine as best you can—without the news.

- **Use your support network**—your friends, your church or place of worship, your own doctor, or your family—for support during transitions like the days after tragedies. These people want and will listen to you.

Tips for Supporting Children Who Remain Scared

- First thing—remember you know your children better than anyone. Before you explain anything or offer up further details or explanations you think your children may need, ask what they have heard, what they have learned, and how it makes them feel. Listen long before you speak. However, know that silence isn't helpful in crises—if your children don't speak about it, open up the conversation and start talking. Continue to ask open-ended questions this week and beyond.

> *Listen long before you speak.*

- Discuss all of the safety measures you take in your own home and at school to protect your children from harm.

- Listen for errors in their understandings so that you can help clear up misinformation and misconceptions. This is something we can do really well!
- If your children don't know about the tragedy, consider talking with them about it prior to returning to school. It's likely a segment of their peers will know about the events of a tragedy or shooting, so it's better for them to hear first about the shooting from you.
- Keep in mind that age really matters here. Children 8 years and younger really don't have an accurate understanding of space and time. Seeing footage from a school may confuse them, or they may believe something scary is happening at their own school. Be really careful when exposing them to any media (TV, printed papers, Internet browsing) that has photos or words they can read.
- Honesty is best. Answer candidly but refrain from gory details. No young child needs to know the age of children who were murdered in a shooting, for example. No young child needs to know the types of weapons or bullets or even the number of children or teachers who died. But children really do want to know how you feel. Talk about what you do to deal with your own sadness or complicated emotions right now. You don't have to know why this happened—it's OK to tell your children you don't know why a tragedy happened.
- In the afternoon/evening after school, check in with your children about their day. Ask open-ended questions to see what they've learned or how they are feeling. Continue to check in over the weeks. These kinds of upsetting experiences are unfortunately far from over on day number 2.

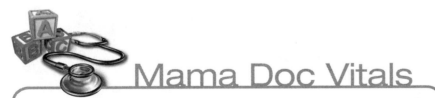

Mama Doc Vitals

Link: HealthyChildren.org link for helping after school shootings: http://bit.ly/mdm-SchoolViolence

Parent Power: It's always OK to say you don't know why something happened.

Tip: If your child is having a difficult time coping with breaking or tragic news, *don't hesitate* to check in with your child's doctor or nurse practitioner. We are trained to help support children and families who are suffering.

16

Less Is More: Pinkeye, Fever, Ear Infections, Teething, and Computed Tomography Scans

Less is more. So often with children, the less we do, the better. Pediatricians often pride themselves on being smart enough to know when to do…nothing.

Pinkeye

Take pinkeye, for example. You know, the gnarly, ooey-gooey, eyes-sealed-shut, yellow-crusty-"sleep"-in-the-eye that never goes away? The highly contagious infection with which your child looks über-crummy and straight-up infectious? When it happens, you create a self-imposed lockdown-blinds-drawn-cancel-all-plans-covert-stay-home and watch a movie to hole up the contagion. You or your child may want to hide from the world until it improves.

In my practice, pinkeye is one of the infections that inspires me to wash my hands over and over and over again. It is really contagious. And the best thing you can do when you see a glimpse of it, anywhere, is wash your hands. But when you have a child with pinkeye, it's different.

So you haul your child in to see the pediatrician. Question is, what does your doctor do for your child? School is asking for a note to come back and you're there for a quick fix, thinking, "Just give me something to make this go away. And fast." And like always, it depends on a number of things.

Your pediatrician will want to determine if the "pinkeye" is caused by a bacterial or viral infection. Studies vary but as a general rule, up to 50% of infections can be viral. So not all need antibiotics. At a glance, it can be hard to tell. Doctors use the history they take, other associated symptoms (runny nose, cough, fever, ear pain), and duration of symptoms to guide them. But without a culture, sometimes it can be difficult to know if a child needs antibiotic drops. And we hate to give antibiotics when we really don't need them. Doctors can turn to some new research to help.

Ways for you to do less (avoid unnecessary visits/medications)…

Four Ways to Know Your Child Is Less Likely to Have a Bacterial Eye Infection

1. Your child is older than 6 years.
2. It's summer! Bacterial infections are less likely between April and November.
3. Your child only has watery discharge (not ooey-gooey yellow/green stuff).
4. Your child is *not* waking up in the morning with "eyes glued shut." If your child wakes up with sealed eyes, call the doctor!

Phew. Now you know. This may help you feel better if the pediatrician suggests not to use antibiotics. Good to know while washing your hands…

Less really is more.

Fever

Every parent talks about fever. It's a hallmark of illness and also the hallmark of parental worry. And I admit that a fever to me as a mom is very different than a fever to me as a pediatrician. The great (but challenging-to-hear news) is that most fevers are mild, go away on their own, and never demand any treatment. Fever phobia is real, meaning that many parents rapidly treat their child's fever with medication when it's often unnecessary. We all get so uneasy when our kids heat up…

So first of all, what is fever?

For most pediatricians, fever is a temperature above 101°F or 101.5°F. But most parents really believe fever starts around 99°F or 100°F, which is by definition an *elevated temperature.* Some infections do cause just a bump in temperature, but others cause real fever. The bottom line is this: pediatricians don't care so much about the number, meaning that it's not that different for us when you tell us that your child has had a temperature of 101°F versus 103°F. No one—moms, dads, children, pediatricians—likes it when a child's fever is above 104°F, but any number under that really might not reflect much of a difference. Clinicians care more about how your child acts, behaves, eats, and plays with fever. And most important in a fever history is knowing how many days a fever has persisted.

> *You want to treat the way your child looks and acts, not what number is on the thermometer.*

So here's the thing about fever: it's protective and may be *productive* for your child when he or she is ill, meaning that when your child has a fever, physiologically the elevated temperature may help get rid of the virus or bacteria that's there. Research has found that some kids with a viral infection who continue to have fever through the course of their illness might recover even faster.

If you decide to treat your child's fever with something like acetaminophen (eg, Tylenol) or ibuprofen (eg, Motrin, Advil), don't treat the number. Your goal is not to go from 103°F to 100°F. Your goal is to take a child who doesn't feel well and make him or her feel better. You want to treat the way your child looks and acts, not what number is on the thermometer.

A Few Fever Rules

- Infants younger than 3 months with fever of any kind or a temperature above 100°F necessitate a trip to see your pediatrician, a call to the nurse, or a trip to an emergency department doctor if it is after hours or when the clinic is closed.
- Fever for up to 3 days can be normal and productive in the face of infection, especially a mild respiratory illness, but if fever is accelerating and rising and not improving over 3 days, you need to check in with your child's doctor.
- **Short-lived Fever:** If your child is otherwise playful, running around the room, and climbing up on chairs, you don't need to treat his or her temperature—you don't need to use acetaminophen or ibuprofen. Furthermore, if you decide to use acetaminophen or ibuprofen, I usually recommend starting with acetaminophen first, as it tends to have fewer side effects like stomach upset or even more serious complications that ibuprofen can have. For healthy children between the ages of 6 months and 12 years, always ask for dosing support if you get confused (see the acetaminophen and ibuprofen dosing chart on page 74).
- When it comes to fever, follow your instincts. If your child looks unwell and you use a fever reducer and your child doesn't look better, call your pediatrician. But know that you don't need to be afraid of fever in and of itself. You really can count on observing your child. Make sure your child is hydrated and getting over the infection as you would expect.

Ear Infections

Ear infections cause significant and sometimes serious ear pain, overnight awakening, missed school, missed work, and lots of parental heartache. For some children, infections in the ear can be a chronic problem and lead to repeated clinic visits, multiple courses of antibiotics, and rarely, a need for tube placement by surgery. For most children, ear infections occur more sporadically, just bad luck after a cold. Fortunately, the majority of children recover from ear infections without any intervention. But about 20% to 30% of the time, they need help fighting the infection.

Ear infections can be caused by viruses or bacteria when excess fluid gets trapped in the middle portion of the ear, behind the eardrum. When that space fills with mucus or pus it is put under pressure and gets inflamed, causing pain. Symptoms of ear infections include pain, fever, difficulty hearing, difficultly sleeping, crankiness, or tugging and pulling at the ear. This typically happens at the time of or soon after a cold; therefore, the fluid in the ear can be filled with a virus or bacteria.

The most important medicine you can give your child when you first suspect an ear infection is one for pain.

Antibiotics only help if bacteria is the cause. When a true infection is present and causing pain and fever, antibiotics are never the wrong choice. Often you'll need a clinician's help in diagnosing a true ear infection.

There's been a lot of work (and research) over the last 15 years to reduce unnecessary antibiotics prescribed for ear infections. There has been great progress. Fewer children see the doctor when they have an ear infection

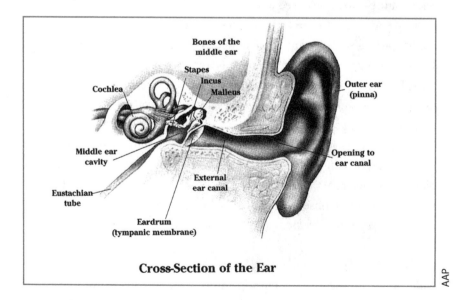

Cross-Section of the Ear

AAP

(only 634 of 1,000 in 2005 versus 950 of 1,000 back in the 1990s) and they're prescribed antibiotics less frequently. Recent data find that fewer than half of children with ear infections receive antibiotics (only 434 of every 1,000 children with ear infections). However, the far majority who go in to see a doctor do still receive a prescription for an antibiotic (76%).

The American Academy of Pediatrics (AAP) released new guidelines early in 2013 to help physicians do a better job treating ear infections. Sometimes children really benefit from using antibiotics, and new research has led to an update of the previously published recommendations. Overuse of antibiotics can lead to more resistant and aggressive bacteria, so we want to use them at the right time. These recommendations may help improve care for children.

In my opinion, NPR published the best article I've read covering the new recommendations. I especially liked the balance provided.

"'When the diagnosis is correct, then antibiotic treatment is never wrong,' says Dr. Ellen Wald of the University of Wisconsin School of Medicine and Public Health in Madison. 'Kids tend to recover more often and they recover more quickly if they're treated appropriately with antibiotics.'

"That's especially important for working parents, Wald notes.

"'We live in a society where there is so much pressure for both parents to be working outside the home and it's just complicated when our child is sick. Besides which, there's always parental anxiety and concern when their child is sick,' she says."

Information for Parents: New Ear Infection Guidelines

- **Pain:** Use medication like ibuprofen or acetaminophen to treat pain when a child has a suspected or confirmed ear infection. These infections really hurt; don't wait for antibiotics to "kick in" or make your child tough it out. On the next page is a summary on dosing pain medications for infants and children.
- **Diagnosis:** The AAP recommendations apply more strict criteria for making the diagnosis of an ear infection. For true diagnosis, the eardrum has to be bulging and there has to be middle-ear fluid or draining fluid from the ear. The ear can't just be red or have a bit of fluid behind it. It's important that the doctor confirm an ear infection before antibiotics are prescribed.
  If a clinician says to you, "It looks like an early ear infection," "The ear drum is a little red," or "I think this may be an ear infection," chances are it doesn't meet criteria and shouldn't be treated with antibiotics. Press the clinician to explain to you if the eardrum is bulging and full of fluid. If there is no proof, antibiotics may not be necessary. Time may be the best medicine.

Weight AGE	8-12 lb. 1-3mo	12-17 lb. 4-11mo	18-23 lb. 12-23mo	24-35 lb. 2-3yrs	36-47 lb. 4-5yrs	48-59 lb. 6-11yrs
Acetaminophen **Infant Drops** 80mg/0.8mL	0.4mL (40mg)	0.8mL (80mg)	1.2mL (120mg)	1.6mL (160mg)	-	-
Acetaminophen **Infant Solution** 160mg/5mL	1.25mL (40mg)	2.5mL (80mg)	3.75mL (120mg)	5mL (160mg)	7.5mL (240mg)	10mL (320mg)
Acetaminophen **Suspension/Solution** 160mg/5mL	-	2.5mL (80mg)	3.75mL (120mg)	5mL (160mg)	7.5mL (240mg)	10mL (320mg)
Ibuprofen **Infant Drops** 50mg/1.25mL	-	1.25mL (50mg)	1.875mL (75mg)	-	-	-
Ibuprofen **Children's Solution** 100mg/5mL	-	-	3.75mL (75mg)	5mL (100mg)	7.5mL (150mg)	10mL (200mg)

Used with permission from The Everett Clinic

Acetaminophen may be given every 4 - 6 hours, not more than 5 times in 24 hours.
Ibuprofen may be given every 6 - 8 hours, usually no more than 3 times in 24 hours.

- **No antibiotics:** Many children don't need antibiotics to heal from ear infections. When a confirmed ear infection is discovered in a child older than 2 years who has no fever or severe ear pain, the child can be observed for 2 days without antibiotics. However, if pain is still present or symptoms have not improved in 48 hours, follow-up is suggested. Make sure you have a good follow-up plan or a prescription written to use if your child isn't improving.

- **Follow-up:** The recommendations remind us that if you choose not to use antibiotics, you need to have a system in place for a follow-up visit, electronic visit, or call in place 48 to 72 hours later. If symptoms of the ear infection resolve in 2 to 3 days with pain medication and time, the ear infection is likely healing. If symptoms (on or off medication) aren't better in 2 to 3 days, your child needs to be seen again to start antibiotics or switch medications.

- **Antibiotics:** All infants younger than 6 months, children 6 to 23 months of age with a double ear infection, those with severe infections, and those at risk for complications need antibiotics. Penicillin (typically amoxicillin—the pink stuff) is the medication used first for ear infections. However, if your child has had amoxicillin in the last month, the clinician should advance the antibiotic (typically to a penicillin with an ingredient called clavulanate to fight resistant bacteria that may be present). Lots of parents worry that amoxicillin isn't the best first choice. Data continue to suggest it is.

- **Eye and ear infection:** If your child has conjunctivitis (pinkeye) or drainage from the eyes along with an ear infection, he or she should immediately get a dose of amoxicillin-clavulanate (Augmentin) rather than amoxicillin (penicillin). Infections that cause both infections (ear and eyes) tend to be more likely to be resistant to amoxicillin.

- **Vaccines:** Immunizations do a good job preventing many ear infections. Make sure your child is up to date on all vaccines, but specifically ensure your child is up to date on *Haemophilus influenzae* type b (Hib), Prevnar 13 (updated pneumococcal vaccine), and an annual flu shot. Prevnar 13 shots and expanded recommendations to use flu shots for all children older than 6 months are attributed in part to decreasing rates of ear infections.

- **Prevention:** Breastfeeding and avoiding cigarette smoke remain data-proven strategies to prevent ear infections in children.

What to Do if Your Child Has a Suspected Ear Infection

- See your pediatrician for an ear check if you are concerned about an ear infection in your child.

- When pediatricians diagnose an infection, push them on the appearance of the eardrum. It's always OK to ask what it looks like! Ask if the eardrum is bulging, has pus behind it, or is red in color. It's OK to ask a pediatrician to clarify and explain the difference between fluid in the ear and an ear infection. In combination with your child's symptoms, it will be important for making a plan.

- If there is difficultly seeing the eardrum, expect the pediatrician to clear earwax from the outside of your child's ear. Hold on. *Remember that seeing the eardrum is the most important part of determining how to help your child.*

- If doctors say it's an "early infection" or "just a bit red" or they are unsure if it's infected, consider asking about avoiding the use of antibiotics. Consider using just pain control and supportive care instead.

- If your child has not improved after 48 to 72 hours from when symptoms started (treated with antibiotics or not), return to see the pediatrician for another evaluation.

Teething

The only medicine I recommend for teething is acetaminophen. The oral teething gels and teething tablets may carry risk. Previously, the US Food and Drug Administration (FDA) released a recall of Hyland's teething tablets. The recall stemmed from concerns of increased and varying amounts of belladonna, a toxic substance that could cause serious systemic effects to babies. It's unclear how much belladonna is found in these tablets normally, although it is well known it's in them. Infants have developed symptoms consistent with belladonna toxicity after using the tablets (change in consciousness, constipation, skin flushing, dry mouth). Homeopathic supplements and medications are unregulated, and therefore it's hard to know what is in them, how consistent one bottle is with the next, and how different brands of the same products compare. Local and national poison control previously deemed teething tablets safe even though it is known that they have trace amounts of belladonna (and possible caffeine). The FDA states it is "unaware of any proven clinical benefit from the product." Because of safety concerns and with no known benefit, I've always recommended against using teething tablets. With my children, I did not and would not use teething tablets. If you have these at home, throw them out. If your child has had these tablets in the past, there is no reason to worry. Ill effects would have been seen soon after using them.

Some Teething Truths

- Teething commences around 4 to 12 months of age and continues until around 24 months, although variability is the norm. Late teethers are very common (first tooth after 9 months) and not worrisome. I recommend you see a dentist after 12 months of age for routine preventive screening. If there are no teeth by 14 to 15 months, that's when a workup (like getting x-rays) would begin.
- Drooling does not necessarily mean your child is teething. Don't let grandparents, neighbors, and friends fool you. Drooling picks up readily after 3 to 4 months of age as a result of your baby's increased exploration by mouth (gnawing and putting hands in mouth) and to facilitate digestion. Prior to a big burst of drool, babies explore through their sense of sight and hearing; as 4 months hits, they start to explore through taste. Although there can be a spike in the volume of drool if a tooth is on its way, it's not a perfect flag for the event.

- Teething discomfort is uncommon. Most babies are utterly unfazed by teeth popping through, while others may show discomfort. *In my office, parents often report the experience of discomfort when their child is teething.* This may be true for some babies, but don't expect to see pain with teething. All babies are different, but research does not associate teething with pain, runny nose, fever, or diarrhea. If your baby has a fever while teething, it's likely from another source (eg, viral infection, ear infection). If your baby has a temperature above 100°F and you are concerned about pain, don't assume it's teething; call or visit your doctor for help.
- When teething, most babies love to chew on things. I often say to parents that it looks like they have itchy teeth! I learned this while watching my boys pop teeth; it really appeared like they wanted to scratch them. But don't misinterpret chewing behavior for pain and reach for medications. You don't have to medicate the urge to gnaw.
- Nearly all babies pop their lower central incisors (2 middle teeth) first, and then the rest of the mouth fills up. Babies get about one tooth per month after their first incisors come in. Order and timing are extremely variable— some babies get one tooth every month, while some infants pop 4 to 6 teeth all at once!
- Teething often causes babies to wake up at night.

Medications Marketed for Teething

1. **Tablets** (homeopathic teething tabs like those recalled): I never recommend these. There's no good evidence that they work. Why give your baby something that potentially can have negative effects with no proven benefit? Regarding homeopathic supplements, The Medicine Guy explains, "The terms dietary, natural, and homeopathic convey a sense of safety. Cultural beliefs, positive reviews from friends, effective selling techniques, and wishful thinking contribute to the impression that a product will be effective for its intended use. Unfortunately, it is not often that we have the clinical evidence to support the effectiveness of most of these products." Furthermore, never rub aspirin or any other medication on your baby's gums.

2. **Gels** (a local anesthetic—usually benzocaine—to numb the gums) like Orajel or Baby Orajel: I don't like these. First of all, if any of you have tried using these, they numb up your mouth, leaving you with a fuzzy, funny feeling inside. They only work on superficial skin, not necessarily targeting the

area of possible discomfort below the gums where teeth are moving. Lastly, I don't like the idea that these gels can potentially numb the back of the throat as they are swallowed by infants, setting a baby up for difficulty swallowing or choking-like behavior.

3. **Liquid pain relievers:** These are the safest and most effective medication for teething. The only medication I ever recommend is acetaminophen (eg, Tylenol). I don't recommend ibuprofen for teething (in my opinion, the risks outweigh the benefit).

If a baby is teething, reach first for symptom relief with teething toys. Then try acetaminophen if you believe your child is in pain.

How to Help Teething Symptoms (Without Medications)

1. **Teething toys:** Find something for your little gnawer that's cool to touch but tough to chew on—a wet washcloth chilled in the freezer for 15 to 30 minutes, a frozen banana or berries if you've introduced solids, solid (not liquid-filled) teething rings chilled in the fridge or freezer (take them out before they are rock hard), a frozen bagel, your finger, or a "lovey"-type toy. If your baby is older than 6 to 9 months, offer a slow-flow sippy cup of cool water to suck on and drink for comfort. Of note, plastic teething rings with liquids have been given a bad name in the past few years due to recalls— potential bacteria growing in liquid and the possibility of a baby cutting through the ring and into the liquid. As many parents try to avoid plastics (due to presence of phthalates/BPA), I suggest using the washcloth method or a cotton sock rolled up tightly to gnaw on. Silicone and latex chewy toys may be a safer bet. One of our boys loved a popular Giraffe teether. And some babies who seem irritated by teething may enjoy having a pacifier to suck on.

2. **Fingers:** Let your baby gnaw on your fingers (if his or her teeth haven't come through), or rub your baby's gums with your clean fingers for comfort.

3. **Massage:** If you're breastfeeding and your baby isn't interested in a teething toy but more interested in chewing on your nipples (eeeeeek) or your arms, especially around the time of feeding, massage your baby's gums with your fingers dipped in cool water prior to starting a feeding.

Clean teething toys, washcloths, or socks after each use. And know that it's absolutely fine to let your baby chew all day if he or she enjoys it. Still, nothing about gnawing means pain.

Pediatric Computed Tomography Scans

Where you get a pediatric computed tomography (CT) scan matters.

After I saw reports of the 5-fold increase in CT scans in children, I asked for my husband's take. I worry about a rise in the use of pediatric CT scans in the United States because when children get scanned, they are being exposed to radiation. A CT scan is a series of x-rays taken in quick succession that form a more composite view of the body. Although x-rays and CT scans save lives and improve diagnosis, the radiation given to children when obtaining these studies must be minimized. Children are more sensitive to radiation than adults; their bodies are still developing. And as the Society for Pediatric Radiology reminds, "What we do now lasts their lifetimes." Here's information on why it may matter where your child gets a CT scan by Jonathan Swanson, MD, a pediatric radiologist at Seattle Children's Hospital.

If it were my child, and Finn or Oden needed to go to an emergency department (ED), I would go to the nearest children's hospital…to spare my children unnecessarily high radiation exposure. *Bias alert: I am a pediatric radiologist working at a children's hospital.* However, I think the literature supports my position.

David Larson, MD, MBA, and colleagues published a paper in *Radiology* in 2011 that confirmed a trend that those of us in the pediatric world have long suspected—the use of computed tomography (CT) scans in children who visit the ED has increased substantially over the last 10 to 15 years. According to their research, from 1995 to 2008, the number of pediatric ED visits that included CT examination increased from 330,000 to 1.65 million, a 5-fold increase. In other words, if your child were to go to the ED today, he or she would be 5 times more likely to have a CT scan than if your child were to be ill back in 1995. Amazing. The older generation of doctors are groaning somewhere, mumbling, "Whatever happened to the physical exam?"

What I find fascinating is that according to this study, 90% of these emergent CT scans occur at adult-focused hospitals, and only 10% occur in children's hospitals. Really? Sure, children's hospitals are not ubiquitous, but I would have thought that more than 10% of families have relatively easy access to a children's hospital. Maybe I am wrong, but my guess is that some of those families who ended up at a community hospital had a choice of a children's hospital and for whatever reason—proximity, ED wait time, advertisement—they chose the community hospital.

According to this study, adult-focused and children's hospitals showed a similar alarming rate in the increased use of CT scans. So choosing a children's hospital may not avoid the CT scan. But this paper suggests, and I agree, that going to an adult-focused hospital when your child needs a CT scan may expose your child to a higher dose of radiation.

Radiation Dose Varies Among Hospitals

- In the study Larson et al write, "Adult-focused facilities may have many competing priorities; focus on pediatric CT may be hard to achieve because of the relatively small volume that pediatric CT represents at such institutions."

- Larson et al cite a 2001 study (Paterson et al) of mostly community-based hospitals that found that CT radiation doses were not typically adjusted for children's smaller body size. In other words, even though lower-dose CT scans on children can provide equal-quality images as full-dose scans on adults, community hospitals did not tend to make the adjustment to the lower dose.

- On the flip side, another study found that CT protocols and scans supervised by pediatric radiologists are routinely adjusted to an appropriate dose for children.

- Even if a pediatric radiologist is in the radiology group at an adult-focused community hospital, it is unlikely, if not impossible, for that individual to be involved in all of the pediatric scans.

Why Children May Get a Higher Dose of Radiation at Adult-Focused Hospitals

- Pediatric hospitals are more comfortable with alternative, lower-dose approaches to common diagnoses. Take appendicitis, for example. At a children's hospital, the first line of imaging for appendicitis is abdominal ultrasound. Ionizing radiation in an ultrasound is zero. In an adult-focused hospital, CT is often the first imaging tool because it can be very difficult to visualize the appendix by ultrasound in young children. If an ultrasound technologist isn't accustomed to working with children, CT may be a more reliable choice.

- When adult-focused facilities take care of children, there can be a level of discomfort. Kids are the exception in the ED, not the rule. From my experience as a radiologist, when physicians are uncomfortable, they tend to order more tests or order a test that will give them the most information, some of which may be more than they need to make the diagnosis. In the world of radiology, this can translate into a higher-than-necessary dose of CT because higher doses can translate into sharper images. We radiologists like our sharper images. The problem is that sharper images don't always translate into improved diagnostic accuracy.

If you don't have a children's hospital nearby, I recommend you urge technicians and radiologists to ensure your child is receiving the lowest dose. The Image Gently Web site is a great resource and an excellent tool kit for working with your community hospital to lower the pediatric CT dose.

We pediatric radiologists need to continue to work with community hospitals to help remove barriers to decreasing the dose for children. We also need to work with manufacturers of CT scanners to make it near impossible to scan a child with an adult dose of radiation.

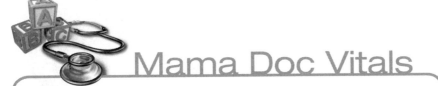

Mama Doc Vitals

Fact: We are exposed to natural, cosmic radiation every day. We get radiation when flying across the country on an airplane too. Each typical cross-country flight gives you the equivalent of about half the radiation you get during a routine 2-view chest x-ray.

Tip: Check out the parent information page at www.imagegently.org for more information. "Children are more sensitive to radiation. What we do now lasts their lifetime."

Parent Power: Speak up if your child receives a CT scan. Ask the physician or technologist to ensure it is the lowest dose possible.

17

Drowning: Quieter and Faster Than You Think

When 2 teenagers died in New York during the summer of 2010, I was shaken. The teens didn't die from a gunshot, a car crash, or suicides. Rather, they drowned in a popular swimming hole in the Bronx River on a hot summer day. I hate stories like that. Hate hearing it, hate seeing the headline. A total failure of prevention efforts.

I talk about drowning in clinic every day I see patients. I should probably talk about it more often. *Drowning is the second-leading cause of injury-related death in children 1 to 19 years of age.* Most drowning in the United States happens during the summer. When it's hot outside, the lake, stream, or pool can look really good. Even to those who don't know how to swim.

I talk about drowning mostly with the parents of toddlers. But I should spend more time talking with adolescents. I get distracted by all the drugs, sex, and rock and roll. The death of those 2 teens still nags on me.

See, drowning isn't what you think it is. It's not loud and splashy and outrageous. It's not like it looks in the movies.

Really, it likely doesn't sound like much at all.

A toddler wanders off, slips in the water, and it's quiet. No noise, no bubbles, no splash.

An adolescent can't keep his chin up long enough and becomes submerged, gradually falling to the bottom of a lake. Quietly.

All this until a family member or friend realizes. Then I think it's really loud.

If we all never let our eyes off our children around the water, and we talk to teens about risks—especially if teens use alcohol around the water (if they drink alcohol and swim, the risks skyrocket)—then maybe you and I can prevent a death. Something we'd never know we did. That's the crazy thing about prevention—it's like an anonymous donation to the world.

- Toddlers drown most often in swimming pools. Even the tiny pools you buy at drugstores or the inflatable pools many of us have.
- Adolescents drown more often in lakes or streams.

- Instincts during drowning are not what you think (the characteristics of what is called the instinctive drowning response). Drowning victims may not look like they are drowning. Drowning victims rarely can call out for help as they struggle. They often can't wave their hands to signal you. Young children may not even have the words to try.

- Young children between the ages of 1 and 4 years are at highest risk for drowning. Never let them out of your sight around water. Even a kiddie pool.

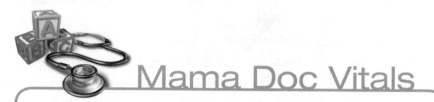

Mama Doc Vitals

Link: Read this incredible perspective called "Drowning Doesn't Look Like Drowning" by Mario Vittone: http://bit.ly/mdm-SilentDrowning.

Fact: Drowning is not as rare as you think. In 2008, 745 children younger than 14 years died from drowning. Eighty-four percent of young children drown at home.

Tip: Have a boy? Make sure safety measures are in place! Boys drown twice as much as girls.

18

Why I Hate the Bouncy House

I hate the bouncy houses. I mean, I really hate them—I get a sick, nervous stomach when the boys are inside them. And it's created a parenting perplexity for me. When I'm at the bouncy houses, I bet my heart rate is about 160 and my blood pressure is 150/90 (translation: high). I'm not kidding—I have a visceral and then flight-type response when the boys jump…it's one of those instinctive parenting responses I am dutifully trying to govern and rule. See, I don't want to hate bouncy houses. I want to be one of those moms who calms down, chats at the sideline, and chills out while my children enjoy the thrill of bounding around a primary-colored, oversized balloon.

I'm not entirely normal on this one. Lots of physicians love those things, and many of our physician friends have bouncy-house birthday parties. A pediatric emergency department doctor I spoke to recently said she gleefully took her son to "the inflatables" too. There was a calm in her voice when she told me. And then envy coming out of mine—I want to simply let my kids enjoy these houses without feeling tortured. But when Finn and Oden are bounding around in one of those houses, big kids flying, and limbs and heads rising about the horizon, I worry. And I can't seem to rid myself of the response. When the birthday party invitation at the bouncy house comes with a waiver of fiscal responsibility for injury or death, you know something is up.

The problem behind the parenting perplexity, ultimately, is that the boys unquestionably love those things. Trouble is, I'm biased; I've taken care of children injured on trampolines and bouncy houses. And I remember a mentor of mine in residency swearing off trampolines; he stated they were an absolute "NO." My husband sees trampoline injuries and fractures all the time. On top of it, when my young boys jump in, they don't have the judgment to steer clear of the big kids or pace/gauge their jumping. It's not that I want them living in a bubble, but a broken neck image turns me instantly to a helicopter mom. "Let kids be kids; lay off, Mom." Right? I unfortunately stand my emotional ground: I don't like them.

Biggest trouble is that data on bouncy house injuries back up my worry. However, the compromise I've made is when the boys go to bouncy houses, we follow a few rules and I stay home. Better for everyone.

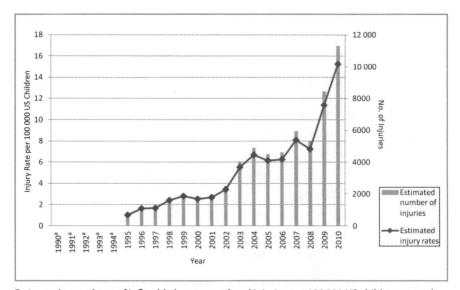

Estimated annual rate of inflatable bouncer–related injuries per 100 000 US children treated in US hospital emergency departments (EDs) and estimated annual number of inflatable bouncer–related injuries to children treated in US hospital EDs, 1995 to 2010.
aNational estimates of annual injury rates and numbers for 1990 to 1994 were not calculated because there were <20 actual cases in each of these years, making estimates unstable.
Source: Thompson MC, Chounthirath T, Xiang H, Smith GA. Pediatric inflatable bouncer–related injuries in the United States, 1990–2010. *Pediatrics*. 2012;130(6):1076–1083

During the 2 decades spanning from 1990 to 2010, nearly 65,000 children were treated for bouncy-house injuries, but as the years unfolded, rates of injuries accelerated. Bouncy-house injuries more than doubled between 2008 and 2010, and most current rates now find that 31 children are treated in emergency departments every day here in the United States for injuries in a bouncy house.

A bouncy-house party place recently closed in Seattle after it filed for bankruptcy, apparently because of lawsuits. So, although the trend to bounce is going up, the future remains a bit murky.

You don't likely hate bouncy houses like I do. So to enjoy them more, here are a few tips to protect your children.

Five Rules to Maximize Safety With Kids in a Bouncy House

- **Make rules ahead of time.** Be clear with your children that when they break the rules, they lose rights to bouncing.
- **Age?** I recommend children younger than 6 years never use trampolines. I don't know what age to tell you about bouncy houses. In my ideal world, I'd say I think preschoolers shouldn't be in them, but reality shows that many preschool parties include these houses and they tend to be a hit! Young children may not have the coordination, skill, or judgment to protect themselves. They need supervision and feedback about their choices while in the houses. Be there and let them know how you experience their choices. Take breaks if kids are getting wild.
- **Try to have children bounce alone or with children of similar age and size.** Nearly 10% of injuries occur from collisions in the bouncer. This may seem challenging in a public or large-party bouncy house! But do your best to avoid having adults or large children bouncing with smaller ones. The weight differential can throw off the bounces, and falls/collisions can be more worrisome.
- **Don't bounce with your children** (see previous point). If you get into the bouncy house, observe from the sidelines. And remember, your standing at the side may not prevent injury (50% occur with parental supervision) but may be a great help to keep children following the rules and understanding the "why" behind them.
- **Use caution by doors and openings in bouncy houses** where children could fall or be injured with the flow of traffic coming and going.

19

Seven Truths About the "Stomach Flu"

We've had our share of "vomitoriums" at our home. Stomach bugs tend to be the nastiest illnesses our children bring home from school. As a mom and pediatrician, here are my 7 truths and tips for survival of stomach bugs when they hit your home.

1. **Hand washing** and keeping things clean are your best defenses from getting ill with a stomach bug. Not surprisingly, this is particularly true after touching or supporting your child and when preparing food and eating. Some viruses will survive on surfaces for days. And some viruses like *Norovirus* can even survive hand sanitizer. You have to use soap and water to kill it. But even with ridiculous, meticulous attention to hygiene, every parent knows that when the vomit is flying, it's hard to lasso every single errant particle. So simply commit to do your best. Change the sheets and clean up areas of vomit immediately after supporting your child. Soapy warm water is your friend. Wash surfaces immediately, use hot water for the wash, and use high heat in the dryer.

2. **24 hours (or so):** In general, most pediatricians will tell you that vomiting doesn't exceed 24 hours with typical gastroenteritis. Occasionally it can. Many kids don't follow the rules. Once a virus that causes gastroenteritis takes hold of a child, vomiting starts. Children tend to vomit more than adults, but I've never read or learned why this is. Part may be an easy gag reflex. With most viruses that cause the "stomach flu," as the infection moves through the stomach and intestines, vomiting stops after about 24 hours. But not always. If you advance liquids too quickly or children eat more solids than they are ready for, even after the first meal 1 to 2 days into eating again, they may have a vomit encore. If you have one of those, start back where you started (sips of clear liquids) and go very slow advancing their diet. If vomiting is accelerating at 24 hours, it is time to check in with your child's doctor.

3. **Disgusting and terrifying:** It's creepy-eepy to take care of a child with vomiting. Not only is it entirely gnarly and disgusting to remove and clean chunks from vomit-laden carpet, sheets, and clothing, it's also terrifying

to provide support to a vomiting child because you can get equally uneasy about catching the virus. You're not alone in this. It's absolutely nauseating to see your own child ill, unwell, and retching. And it's awful to imagine having to provide care while getting miserably sick. Do your best to keep your hands washed and keep the love going. As all of us know, when you find yourself picking out vomit bits from the carpet at 3:00 am, it really can only get better from there.

4. **Medication:** Children rarely need medication when recovering from gastroenteritis. Although some antinausea drugs are available for use in children, most children don't need prescription medications. Talk with your child's pediatrician if you feel you child is vomiting longer than 24 hours or becoming dehydrated. Remember that vomiting is a protection reaction of your child's body to clear infection.

5. **Soap, water, and bleach:** I was reminded today that William Osler said, "Soap and water and common sense are the best disinfectants." Cleaning your home to avoid spreading infection is a must. You don't need expensive products, just vigilance. With some highly infectious viruses that cause vomiting, even 10 viral particles can cause illness. So in addition to soap and water, consider using a dilute bleach solution to clean hard surfaces.

Many household bleach products are now registered with the Environmental Protection Agency (EPA), and on the EPA Web site (http://bit.ly/mdm-PPLS) you can look up product-specific dilutions. For example, for some products, the "formula" is ½ cup of bleach per gallon of water for disinfecting or 2 teaspoons per gallon for sanitizing (but check the labels or the EPA Web site to be sure).

6. **Detective work:** Sometimes you'll simply never know where it all came from. But it won't stop you from playing the role of infectious detective. Literally, I have caught myself daydreaming about the moment that the viral particles have entered my little boy's body. How I'd love to return to that moment and intervene against the germs, those little gremlins. The only issue: this is simply wasted time.

7. **Yummy, clingy love:** There is an occasional perk to a terrible stomach bug. And we have to find one to maintain a sense of optimism. When our children are ill, they really turn over and show us they want us over anything

else on earth. Sometimes, my good friend Dr Claire says, "We're magic too." And I totally agree—there is an intimacy that rises in illness. I nicknamed Oden "Velcro" during a recent bout of vomiting. He simply wouldn't leave my side…magic.

Then there is resilience. Children do very well recovering from typical viral gastroenteritis, although diarrhea can last for days. Even so, our children's resilience will long astonish us.

Feeding a Child When Recovering From Stomach Bugs

- Children should go very slow drinking liquids after vomiting. Don't trust your 3-year-old to know how to pace taking in liquids. Offer sips slowly. Start with clear liquids, preferably something with electrolytes (eg, Pedialyte) due to lower sugar content, and water, broth, or very dilute juice. Start with sips every 10 minutes or so for just a few ounces of liquid an hour.
- Once your child has tolerated sips for about 6 hours, consider a bland, boring food. Think of things without extra fats like salty crackers, bread, noodles, or rice. After your child has had a few hours of tolerating those foods, allow more volume and more complex foods. Remember, continue to go slow advancing back to your child's typical diet. There's always a possibility for a barf encore, so be careful. You don't necessarily need to avoid cow's milk, but I wouldn't start with it.
- For infants, human milk or formula are best for feeding. Infants don't need juice or even electrolyte solution in most cases.

When to Call the Doctor

If you're at all concerned about dehydration due to a lack of tears with crying or minimal urine output in your child's diaper or on the toilet, or you see very chapped, dry lips or dry mouth, call your child's doctor for advice or a visit.

If your child has a persistent high fever, is complaining of abdominal pain, or hasn't had any liquids for more than one day, you may need an urgent visit for an evaluation. Trust your instincts and call the office when necessary.

Mama Doc Vitals

Tip: One of the biggest ways that *Norovirus* is transmitted is through contaminated food. Don't prepare food while you're ill or for 3 days after you've had the "stomach flu."

Tip: Bleach solution: Mix between 15 and 25 tablespoons of bleach in 1 gallon of water. Use this bleach water solution to clean the bathroom, counters, and toys. Don't hesitate to mix it up and re-clean the day after you and your child are improved, as your child's poop will likely still contain some of the very contagious virus particles. Wash all clothes in a long washing cycle and then use a dryer to further kill potential virus that remains.

Parent Power: When you and your children are ill, take slow sips of fluids throughout the day to keep your fluids up. Don't give your children a sippy cup or water bottle full at first—often a big amount of liquid at once will come right back up! Think spoonfuls.

New Bike

Wonder all mixed up with dread, Finn got a new bike over a holiday weekend when he was 5 years old. Great trepidation on my behalf spun into sincere pride. For Finn, it was just another joy, another leap into the chapters of requisite or quintessential childhood. To Finn, the transition to the bike seemed to feel fresh and cool, like dipping his toes into a new stream. Although I saw fear in his eyes for small moments while on the bike, most of the time his face was immediately lit with exhilaration. When he spun his pedals it really looked as if he felt he was flying. Allowing those wings to unfold is the privilege and pleasure of parenting. Trouble is, the new bike came with a bit of dread—for me, mostly; a little bit for Finn. Although he puttered around on a balance bike for a year prior, the new bike afforded an enormous transition. We're talking hard metal, big wheels, shimmering blue paint, and pop-a-wheelie potential. This was the real-deal bicycle, the kind that goes on roads with lines down the middle and can take him to the park. It turns out my little boy was growing up. Enter dread, stomach drop, and delight all over again and all at once.

Sometimes I think my worry comes from my work. I have seen, and continue to see, many children with injuries from bicycles. I suppose seeing them, caring for them, and hurting for them alongside their parents colors my sense of vulnerability. I must say, I simply didn't expect to feel so fragile with his bike. When we headed to the bike store late on a Saturday afternoon, I had no idea we were crossing a line in the sand.

A new era—all of the sudden I had this big kid, this big road, and this big opportunity. Yes, in my brain I was certain this was good for Finn and Oden; it was my heart that was catching up.

After clinic, the boys and I used to spend the evenings at a local park cruising around on the trails and peddling under a big blue sky. As Mount Rainier loomed over us and the sun cast its sideways light, we found ourselves sneezing amid the shrubs and vegetation. We played hide-and-seek and tumbled on the ground after laying our bikes along the path. This wasn't our typical Tuesday. And as my fondness grew for the bike, I was reassured that this new chapter (boys with bikes) was a luxurious one that stretches our margins, expands our boundaries, and creates profound potential. New places await us.

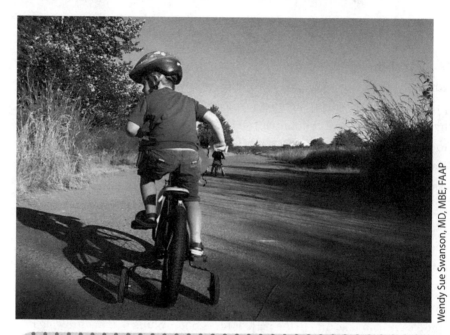

Wendy Sue Swanson, MD, MBE, FAAP

It dawned on me—think of fitting a helmet like finding a perfect bra; it has to fit in all directions, and all the straps should be snug but not too snug.

But to keep this life-chapter from turning into a page-turner, I'll steady myself and talk about helmets. Layering safety protection often dampens my fear and helicopter-mama anxieties. The helmet is the perfect accessory for my panic-like first-time-mom-with-2-sons-on-bikes transition.

Because children are severely injured on bicycles every year, one thing we all know to do is go out and get a helmet for our kids. More important may be making sure the helmet fits. It's not as easy as you would imagine. Poorly fit helmets are biking around you all the time. So don't use your neighbors as an example. After getting Oden a new helmet, I had to check my facts.

It dawned on me—think of fitting a helmet like finding a perfect bra; it has to fit in all directions, and all the straps should be snug but not too snug.

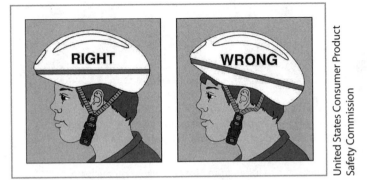

Figure 22.1.

Fitting a Bike Helmet

- **Timing:** Fit the helmet before you pull out the bike. The toe tapping, tugging to get out the door, and true sense of urgency won't be there, and you'll find time to get it fit properly. Better yet, fit it with your child inside and then show the results.
- **Eyes:** Your child should be able to see the helmet without a mirror! Have your child confirm this by looking up when the helmet is on. The helmet has to be squarely situated on the forehead, about 2 fingers' widths above your child's eyebrows. You really want it to rest down on your child's forehead, fitting more like a helmet and less like a ball cap or a yarmulke. If the helmet isn't snug on the forehead, when a child falls forward on the pavement, for example, it won't protect the skull from the front when he or she hits (negating the point of wearing it altogether).
- **Ears:** Your child's ears should be framed by a Y strap (Figure 22.1). I think this may be the most difficult part when adjusting a helmet because you often have to pull the straps from all directions. Take your time. Try again when necessary. Make sure the ear rests just above the Y and that the straps are snug against the side of your child's face.
- **Mouth/jaw:** Although mastering the Y strap may be most difficult for you, the chin strap may be most difficult for your child. You want the chin strap to be snug enough to help keep the helmet in place in case of a crash on the ground. You want about one finger's width of space between the chin and the strap with the mouth closed. When your child opens his or her jaw to scream, yell, or chew, it should tug on the helmet from above. The strap should be snug but never so snug that it leaves a mark on the skin after wearing it.

Mama Doc Vitals

Tip: Bike helmets with the CPSC sticker are certified and safe for biking but not for rollerblading, roller-skating, or skateboarding (ASTM 1492 sticker). Look for dual-certified safety stickers if your child is going to use it for all types of activities.

Fact: Wearing a helmet reduces injury from bike and bike-motor vehicle accidents more than 80% of the time.

Tip: Take the helmet off at the park or playground. The straps can get stuck or snagged on equipment and cause your child to choke or have difficulty breathing.

21

Helicopter: You Betcha

When we took the training wheels off of Finn's bike, my heart surely skipped a few beats. Mind you, Finn never really needed the training wheels, as he'd already learned how to balance on 2 wheels with his balance bike as a toddler. Yet somehow he decided he wanted them on and that it would be a more enjoyable transition if he got to use them. Trouble was, once on, it was difficult to convince him he didn't need them. And it was difficult for me to want to unscrew them. The morning we finally took them remains vivid in my mind: the sun cast gorgeous light over Seattle and we realized there were 2 days left of summer in the Pacific Northwest. So my dear husband proclaimed it was time: "No more trainers." Finn and I waited nervously at the pavement edge as the Allen wrench was applied.

As I said, I was terrified of that bike. I worried about speed, my loss of control over major injuries and big falls for my little boy, and the greater transition to him biking off and away from home. Something about a big-boy bike felt like an emblematic diploma. It was as if I was granting him permission to grow up. I was dragging my feet.

I knew there are blessings in injuries for children—learning margins for error, witnessing the consequences of ill attention, and the reality that scabby knees are a part of a normal, active childhood. So easy to say as a doctor; so hard to feel as a mom.

Helicopter parent? You betcha. At least a little part of me.

I really don't care what you call me (OK, I do on some level). But know I have distaste for the labeling of parenting "styles" and decision-making, particularly when it enters the research world. I hated the 2011 media blitz on the study describing the risks surrounding "helicopter parents" and obesity. I mean, come on. All this categorizing doesn't really help us. I may be "helicopter" with this decision and then absent-minded, laissez-faire mother with the next; attachment parent on Tuesday; and the cry-it-out champion Friday night.

When it comes to safety, it's imperfect if we hover. Children do need to learn how to self-regulate and learn from their errors, but watching out for broken bones is something I'm still committed to. I realize that as the boys get older, the scope of this injury prevention only increases. I remember reading a blog post from The Teen Doc in which she talks about keeping your hands on your lap while watching the accident happen. She describes the perils and terror of teaching your teen to drive. Thank goodness I have some 11 more years to prepare. Better to ease into these things.

Understanding Risks for Sudden Infant Death Syndrome

New research helps clarify ways we can reduce risks for sudden infant death syndrome (SIDS) or sudden unexplained death in infancy. An April 2012 *Pediatrics* study found that the convergence of risks (Figure 24.1) for infants is meaningful—reducing the number of risks may reduce SIDS deaths. Avoiding multiple and simultaneous SIDS risks may help, especially for babies who are vulnerable due to family history, genetics, prematurity, or prenatal exposures. Further, research published the same year in the *American Journal of Public Health* confirms that sleep environment hazards (co-sleeping, soft sleeping surfaces, shared sleep surfaces with people or animals) contribute to SIDS.

Triple Risk Model for Understanding SIDS Risks

Critical Period of Development

<2 months
2–4 months of age

Extrinsic Risks

Sleep position
Soft bedding
Face covered
Bed sharing
Over-bundling

Intrinsic Risks

Genetics
Prematurity
Male gender
Prenatal exposure to
alcohol/cigarette smoke

Figure 24.1. Triple risk model for understanding SIDS risks.

Seventy percent of infants who died from SIDS were sleeping in a surface not intended for infant sleep (eg, adult bed, couch, chair), and 64% of infants who died were sharing a sleep surface, with half sharing with an adult. We can decrease SIDS risk by controlling our baby's environment, knowing our baby's vulnerabilities, and sharing what we know. Put babies on their backs without soft bedding (bumpers/pillows/blankets) in their own crib until 1 year of age.

The triple risk model helps explain the convergence of risk and reminds parents the part of risk that we can control.

The 2012 study came out looking at the different risk factors and the different types. It used what the authors call the triple risk model; the idea is that when it comes to sudden infant death, we think there are 3 different areas of risk.

One is *family history, genetics, or prenatal exposures.* For example, we know babies exposed to cigarette smoke and alcohol in utero, with a family history of SIDS, and who are born prematurely and are boys are at higher risk for SIDS.

Two is *timing.* We also know that a baby's age is part of that concern or risk. So we know that we only diagnose SIDS when kids are between birth and 1 year of age, but we also know there are critical periods for SIDS during development—it's more common between 1 and 4 months of age. We want families to really decrease other risks during this time.

Third are the *extrinsic factors* or the *environmental factors and risk.* These risks are like where your baby sleeps and on what surface, who's in the bed, and who's with your baby. Is there a blanket there? Is your baby on his or her back? Does your baby have a pacifier in his or her mouth?

What research is starting to demonstrate is that the convergence of all 3 of those risks is helping us understand how to reduce SIDS. What we know is that since we've been putting babies on their back, 50% fewer babies are dying from SIDS every year, and that's incredible. But what we want to know is how can we reduce risks even further.

The 2012 study found that 90% of babies who passed away from SIDS had at least one risk. More than half of babies had at least 2 extrinsic risks and one intrinsic risk. And what we also know is that of the babies who passed away, only 5% had no extrinsic risks at all. That means 95% of babies who died from SIDS died in an unsafe sleep environment. So as parents, what we can do is really control the sleeping environment for our babies and provide them the least risk.

What parents can do to reduce risk for SIDS

- Put babies on their backs in a bare crib at bedtime.
- Put babies to sleep with a pacifier if your babies like that.
- Make sure there's no soft bedding around—no bumpers (including mesh bumpers), pillows, stuffed animals, or loose blankets.
- Make sure there are no cigarette smokers in the house.
- If you're co-sleeping, make sure you're reducing any soft bedding around the baby, reducing the number of parents in the bed (if co-sleeping, no more than 1 adult), and keeping the bed the most bare, alone environment you can for your baby.

WendySueSwanson MD @SeattleMamaDoc

I don't recommend using baby monitors to track baby breathing. No good data they prevent SIDS. Lots of anecdotes they inc parent anxiety.

Why I Hate Sleep Positioners

I hate infant sleep positioners. They are not safe or helpful. If you have one or know a family or friend who uses one for an infant, throw it out. Trash compact it. Stomp on it. Cut it up in bits. This is one rare thing you should feel good about putting in a landfill.

When I first started in practice, I didn't even know sleep positioners existed; I was shocked at how many parents told me they were using them. We are led to believe (by manufacturers) that positioners confer safety by keeping babies on their backs. Since 1994, the Back to Sleep campaign has helped parents become vigilant (yes!) about putting babies to sleep on their backs. But after my sons were born, while roaming the superstore aisles for bottles, crib sheets, overpriced silicon, and breast pads (oh the glory), I realized why parents get so confused.

> *When asked about setting up a safe infant crib, I say, "Boring, bare, basic."*

In the infant sleep section, I found plenty of products designed for babies I would never recommend. Never. Sleep positioners, head positioners, comforter-like blankets for the crib, bumpers, and stuffed animals. Many products went against what I was taught in my pediatric training and what I've learned thereafter. Like so many things in life and medicine, less is more. When asked about setting up a safe infant crib, I say, "Boring, bare, basic."

In 2011, the American Academy of Pediatrics (AAP) issued an updated guideline on preventing SIDS. The AAP has had to reiterate its position citing the dangers of sleep positioners after the US Consumer Product Safety Commission and Food and Drug Administration sent out a warning. Even though these positioners go clearly against safety data and medical advice, companies have kept them on the market.

Why?

Fear. Plenty of products designed for infant sleep target those parents who fear sudden infant death syndrome (SIDS). Which, to be honest, is most of us. Products like sleep positioners claim to keep babies on their backs yet go entirely against what we know in protecting infants from unexplained death or SIDS.

The bad news: SIDS, although extremely rare, is the number one killer of infants beyond the neonatal period.

The good news: Over the past decade and a half, since pediatricians and providers have advised placing babies on their backs to sleep, the rate of SIDS has been cut in half. Getting rid of a positioner is one change that could prevent an avoidable death. A positioner is made of soft bedding material. Boring, sparsely decorated cribs with firm mattresses are the preferred, perfect sleeping environment for babies.

Boring, bare, basic is best.

When you leave the hospital, you need very few material goods: breast milk (or formula), a bare crib or bassinet (with a firm mattress), diapers and wipes, a few outfits, and thin receiving blankets. And the nonmaterial one: love. That comes naturally.

The causes of SIDS are poorly understood. The following information is not to scare you but rather to inform you of ways to minimize the risk:

Preventing Sudden Infant Death Syndrome

- **Position:** Always put your baby to sleep on his or her back. Remember, since the 1990s when we advised back sleeping, death from SIDS has been cut in half. There is no questioning this. Always put a baby to sleep on her back. If your baby rolls over after you've placed her on her back, there is no need to continue repositioning her.
- **People:** Tell grandmas, babysitters, nannies, and the nice friend who helps you out to always put your baby to sleep on her back. Babies who are used to sleeping on their backs and then are placed on their tummies by a different caregiver are at a far increased risk of SIDS.
- **Bedding:** Avoid soft bedding, sleep positioners, head positioners, bumpers, stuffed animals, thick blankets, or pillows of any kind in the first year. Talk with your pediatrician if you have any concerns or want to clarify. Boring, bare, basic.

- **Lifestyle:** Babies who have parents who smoke are at increased risk for SIDS; avoid cigarette smoke and help loved ones quit. Your baby is the perfect reason.
- **Pacifier:** Pacifiers have been shown to decrease the likelihood of SIDS (the why behind this recommendation is debatable). Offer a pacifier to your baby after 1 month of age when feeding is well established. If the pacifier falls out during the night, there are no data to support your need to put it back in a baby's mouth. (Just try to get some sleep!)
- **Cool:** Don't jack up the thermostat because there is a baby at home. Ideal temperature for sleeping infants is about 65°F to 68°F. New data suggest that using a fan to circulate air (not directly on the baby) may improve the condition as well. Keep the room cool. In the summer, use a circulating fan to keep the room comfortable.
- **Where:** The AAP recommends that babies sleep in their own crib or bassinet in their parent's room until 6 months of age. This makes overnight feeding easier too (quick commute).
- **Inform:** Know the facts so you don't make false assumptions and increase your worry. Share what you know.

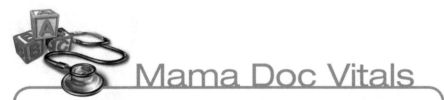

Mama Doc Vitals

Fact: Sudden infant death syndrome (SIDS) is rare but more common in infants who have a family member who died of SIDS or parents who smoke. It is most common between 2 and 4 months of life with 90% of cases occurring in babies younger than 6 months.

Tip: Bare crib until first birthday. Follow precautions and back-to-sleep positioning until your infant turns 1 year of age.

Tip: I recommend against using any kind of bumper, including the mesh bumpers. There are concerns about safety and no data to show any benefit!

Two Is the New One: Rear-Facing Car Seats Until at Least Age 2

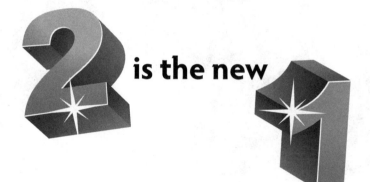

is the new

This is kind of like, "Brown is the new black." But different and more important.

Two is the new one. When you're a toddler. And when you're at least 20 pounds.

And you're in the car.

Even though we have been urging parents to keep children rear-facing in the car until at least 2 years of age, studies find that the majority of parents switch their children prior to their second birthday.

Listen up and tell your friends. Scream from the rooftops. There is good news and bad news to this story.

> *Your small little love is 75% less likely to die or incur a serious injury if rear-facing when riding in the car.*

The bad news first, of course—you're not going to be advised to turn your little 1-year-old forward-facing in the 5-point car seat until he or she is 2 years of age. Yes, yes, I know, you did that with your other child. So did I. I didn't know any better. We evolve, science moves forward, new findings surface. And we now realize that facing-forward is a no-good right of passage for a 1-year-old.

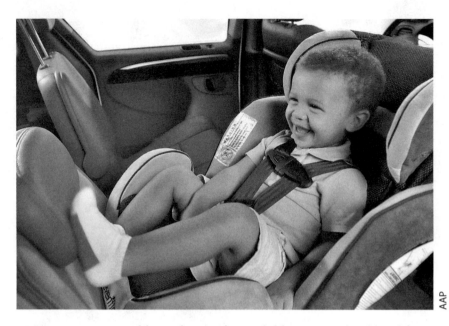

AAP

Keep your 1-year-old rear-facing. If your child is 15 months old and facing the front of the car, go into your car and turn that seat back around. Let go of that dream of doing air high fives in the rearview mirror with your 18-month-old.

Your small little love is 75% less likely to die or incur a serious injury if rear-facing when riding in the car.

Gasp.

Newer guidelines recommend that all children face the rear until age 2. Even if their legs hit the back of the seat. The rationale: children are 5 times safer in rear-facing seats in this age group. Marilyn Bull, MD, FAAP, reviewed studies completed by her team of researchers and the American Academy of Pediatrics recommendations. She says that we rarely, if ever, see spine injuries in children in rear-facing car seats. She continued, "We will see head injuries or we will see a few other injuries, but the vast majority of serious injuries occur when children are forward-facing." To form these opinions, she used data from a study that evaluated the US National Highway Traffic Safety Administration vehicle crash database in children younger than 2 years from 1988 to 2003.

Here's the good news: Your beloved little babe is 5 times safer in a car crash while riding rear-facing when between 12 and 24 months of age than if you flipped him forward-facing.

Five times safer. Seventy-five percent less likely to die or have a serious injury.

Turn your baby around. This is one of those rare no-brainers. There aren't many of those out there anymore.

Some Science and Rationale

- When you stop quickly or are involved in an impact, your body continues to fly forward at the velocity the car was going. This sounds like an eighth-grade math word problem; it isn't. Infants and toddlers have disproportionately big heads for their necks and bodies (read: bobbleheads) so as the car slows, their heads and upper neck continue to move forward rapidly while the straps of the car seat hold their bodies in place. This motion puts them at risk for cervical spine and severe neck injuries.

- When rear-facing, the head, neck, and entire body can absorb the impact at once. This rear-facing position can prevent neck injuries leading to paralysis or even death.

So, we were wrong a few years back to say it was OK to turn your baby around when she was 20 pounds and 1 year old.

Two (years) really is the new one (year).

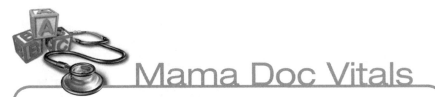

Mama Doc Vitals

Tip: No rush to forward: If a 3- or 5-year-old's seat allows for a child to stay rear-facing, there is no rush to turn the child around. Even if the child's legs hit the back of the seat. Rear-facing in a seat that accommodates a child is always safer.

Fact: Every transition you make with seats—from infant seat, to booster seat, to seat belt in the back seat, to seat belt in the front seat at age 13—decreases protection for your child riding in the car.

Parent Power: Get a car seat safety check if you're concerned about how the seat fits in your car. The Web site www.seatcheck.org will locate the closest location.

Tip: A tip from my friend Alanna Levine, MD, FAAP: Put a mark on the wall at 4' 9" high, the height required to move from a booster seat to a seat belt. As your child ages and enters school and asks to ditch the booster seat, you can always say, "Are you above that line?"

25

Can We Prioritize Sleep?

I wonder—can we prioritize sleep? I mean this sincerely. Can we really value it? Sleep is one of the essential parts of being human, yet unlike some of the other essential things (think food, exercise, oxygen, or shelter), no one seems to give us credit when we sleep. Come about age 11, kids start to be praised for their achievements more than their skills in self-preservation.

Like most busy moms, I speak from an experienced place—I'm often up early after going to bed late. When the dog awakens us with vomiting at 2:30 am, I clock in fewer than 6 hours of sleep as the alarm clock breaks the silence of the morning. Clearly it is our own responsibility to find ways to prioritize sleep. No one will do it for us. So, how we model sleep and also advise our children as they grow matters. It is well understood that sleep deprivation isn't good for us. It's not good for our performance, our driving, our friendships, our mood, or even our waistlines.

In clinic, I ask teenagers what time they go to bed. I ask them if they sleep with their phones, if they wake up to an alarm, and how easy it is to fall asleep. I ask parents, and I ask about the little ones too. But it's the teens (and parents) I worry about most. Those little 6-month-old midnight screamers, they'll figure it out. The oversubscribed, stressed out, high- (or low-) achieving teens? They need a little time on this…

After I ask about bedtime, I ask teens how late they sleep on the weekend. The reason: I want to know about their sleep debt. Sleep debt is the cumulative amount of sleep below what you need. If you needed 8½ hours and you only got 6, you created a 2½-hour sleep debt. It adds up, a lot like any other kind of debt. Fortunately, you can pay it back a bit by making up for it with long periods of rest in the future, taking a nap, or long nights of sleep on the weekend. But I wonder how you do all week while tired. The study evaluated this.

Teens' sleep debt is often high—a 2006 US poll found that nearly a quarter of all teens fall asleep at school. In one report, only 15% of teens said they got more than 8 hours of sleep during the week. If you go to bed around 11:00 pm and school starts at 7:00 am, it's nearly impossible to get what you need. *Teens need about 8½ to 9½ hours a sleep each night.* Part of my job as a pediatrician is to help teens understand that their sleep debt is a sign they aren't getting enough sleep midweek. And it's my job to help motivate them to prioritize sleep. That's the hard part.

Sufficient sleep during adolescence is important for the development of psychosocial functioning, behavioral maturation, and cognition.

In my practice, sleep debt is nearly universal. Most teens report a fair amount of makeup/catch-up/refill-the-tank sleep on the weekend. Do you? I remember crashing on the weekends in high school, college, medical school, and residency. Since my boys have been around—yes, this period of life is sleep-deprived, too—it seems that there is no time when parenting young children for making up sleep! Sleep deprivation has been a huge part of life for me in completing what I needed to do to succeed professionally. So I'm not a great example. Neither is our American culture in general.

> *Sufficient sleep during adolescence is important for the development of psychosocial functioning, behavioral maturation, and cognition.*

When school starts, I'll keep talking to teens about prioritizing sleep like they prioritize food, exercise, friendship, sports, or good grades. I don't know how much good I do, though. Culturally, we seem to have it all a little backwards. We often praise those who perform on 4 hours of sleep. We marvel at surgeons who stay up all night and operate the following day. We commend kids who oversubscribe to activities so that they are left doing homework in the dark. We focus on work ethic. We focus on achievement. We forget to prioritize sleeping and self-care. We don't praise those kids who sleep 9 hours at night. How do we illuminate the cost of sleep deprivation? Science…

A 2011 study found that teens who created a sleep debt throughout the week had a more difficult time performing tests requiring concentration and attention during the week. In a study conducted in Korea, investigators studied more than 2,600 teens and found

- Teens slept an average of 5 hours and 42 minutes a night during the week. Let me just say, that's a failing grade in the sleep department!
- Teens slept an average of 8 hours and 24 minutes on the weekend. They had an average of about 2½ hours of catch-up sleep to restore their debt.

- Teens who had increased hours of catch-up sleep on the weekend had more errors on tasks that required their attention.
- More, they found that increased sleep debt predicted poorer performance on tasks demanding attention more than the number of hours of sleep a child got each night during the week.

So asking kids about sleep debt is a good start. Sleeping late on the weekends may be a flare that a child will have a harder time in school during the week than we knew and that they are at risk for other consequences of sleep deprivation.

WendySueSwanson MD @SeattleMamaDoc

Startling number of school-age children don't get enough sleep. 73% of 9-10 yo tired on test day. US tops the list: bbc.in/10FkKd3

Mama Doc Vitals

Information: Teen sleep information from the National Sleep Foundation: http://bit.ly/mdm-TeenSleep

Study: Research finds that increased weekend catch-up sleep is an indicator of insufficient weekday sleep and is associated with poor performance on objective attention tasks. Translation: even if your teens sleep in until 12:00 noon on Saturday, they aren't getting enough sleep during the week, and their ability to perform at school suffers!

Numbers: Teens need 9¼ hours of sleep each night to function best! If they are up at 6:00 am, that means they should be in bed ideally around 9:00 pm.

Parent Power: The best way to protect your teen's sleep may to push for later start times at school. Check out information around the country for later start times: http://schoolstarttime.org.

26

If It Were My Child: No Texting and Driving

Warning: this is a rant. Recently, when I was driving in front of Seattle Children's Hospital, I saw a car going more slowly than I'd expected, changing the traffic patterns. We stopped at the light, it turned green, and she didn't move. I looked over and saw her punching away at her phone, composing a text message. I laid on the horn. I pointed to her phone. I screamed! She looked surprised and confused that she'd done anything dangerous. I think she wondered why I was so fanatical.

You're 23 times more likely to have a crash while texting and driving compared with someone who is driving without distraction. I wish I could have mentioned that too.

No one was hurt; no one was injured that morning. Yet it appeared the last thing this driver was thinking about was the road, the traffic light, and the children and their parents crossing at the walk while entering and leaving the hospital. Imagine.

> *You're 23 times more likely to have a crash while texting and driving compared with someone who is driving without distraction.*

Texting while driving was responsible for 16,000 deaths in a 6-year period. More than 5,000 lives were lost in 2009 alone and almost half a million people were injured in accidents related to distracted driving.

You know what I mean though, right? You can spot those texters on the road. We've all been behind someone on a side street or the freeway watching the car swerve, veer, or not follow traffic flow. Or think about the drivers who turn abruptly without using a turn signal. And when we look over, we see they're on the phone or punching away at a keyboard. Often, these insidious choices are obvious and for all to see.

If you think you're a fantastic multitasker, think again. Texting and driving kills.

I've had it with people who are still using their phones to text and drive at the same time. Oprah and I couldn't agree more: *end distracted driving now.*

I don't think fear works, and unfortunately a ranting chapter in my book may not be a perfect strategy either. It's possible that focusing on safety isn't the answer. As one pediatric safety researcher said to me, "Maybe there is something psychologically protective in not worrying about safety all the time." She went on to postulate that talking about safety may not be the best angle to take to improve this. That spending our energy on figuring out what factors actually do impact behavior may be better (changing normative beliefs or law-enforcement fines).

Yes, worrying all the time isn't so good for us either.

I contend that texting and driving is a new inconvenient truth; distracted driving is a selfish, dangerous, and morally unjust act. You simply put others (in and out of your car) at risk. Data from 2009 studying real drivers back up my claim. The Virginia Tech Transportation Institute studied the effect of distracted driving using naturalistic driving studies (sophisticated cameras and instrumentation in vehicles) with drivers in cars and trucks on the outcome of a crash or near-crash event. They studied drivers for more than 6 million miles of driving. Here's the skinny.

When in a truck,

- You're 23.2 times more likely to crash or have a near-crash event if you're texting and driving.
- You're 6.7 times more likely to risk a crash or near crash if you're using or reaching for an electronic device.
- You're 5.9 times more likely to risk a crash or near crash if you're dialing a cell phone.

When in a car,

- You're 2.8 times as likely to risk a crash or near crash if dialing a cell phone.
- You're 1.3 times as likely to crash if talking on or listening to a cell phone.
- You're 1.4 times as likely to crash if you're reaching for an object.

By the data, targeting texting may be the effort most necessary. Researchers clearly point out that cell phone use on its own isn't nearly as dangerous. The reason, they feel, is that the results "show conclusively that a real key to significantly improving safety is keeping your eyes on the road." Cell phone use (with voice activation) doesn't interfere with it. Grabbing for your ringing cell phone does. As does texting. When subjects were texting while driving, they had the longest duration of time with eyes off the road (4.6 seconds). "This equates to a driver traveling the length of a football field at 55 mph without looking at the roadway."

Is that beep or buzz of your phone enough to cause you to reach for it while barreling down the road?

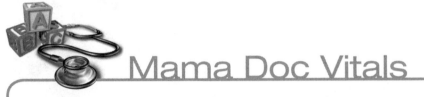

Mama Doc Vitals

Tip: Get in the habit of putting your cell phone/purse/bag in the back seat when you get in the car. Force yourself to refuse that buzz/beep while on the road.

Fact: 45% teens from all over the United States said they had texted and driven during the last month in a 2013 Centers for Disease Control and Prevention report.

Parent Power: Have "house driving rules" and stick to the rules and consequences. There are some data that these rules combined with parent enforcement can reduce risky teen driving behaviors and crashes.

How Do Doctors Screen for Autism Spectrum Disorders?

Pediatricians, nurse practitioners, and family doctors start screening your baby or toddler for signs of developmental or communication challenges like autism spectrum disorders (ASDs) from the very first visit. As a pediatrician, how your baby responds to you (and to me) during the various visits during infancy and toddlerhood guides me in his screening. In the office I get to observe how your baby giggles, how he looks to his parents for reassurance, how he tries to regain mom's attention during our conversation, how he points or waves, how he responds to his name, and even how and why he cries when I'm around. Those observations in combination with family history, health examinations, and parental perspectives remain extremely valuable for me in helping identify children at risk for ASDs.

However, more formalized screening is recommended at the 18- and 24-month well-child checks. In most offices, clinicians use the Modified Checklist for Autism in Toddlers (M-CHAT), a 23-point questionnaire filled out by parents. Often, I have to help parents answer one question in particular ("Does your child make unusual finger movements near his/her face?"), but other than that, most families find it easy to fill out. Using this standardized screening, pediatricians can pick up children at risk for ASDs and will be prompted to start conversations about language delay, concerns about behavior, or possible next steps for a toddler at risk with additional genetic, neurologic, or developmental testing.

It's important to note that screening isn't diagnosing. If your child has a positive screen for an ASD, it doesn't mean he will be diagnosed on the spectrum. And further, if your child screens normally but you continue to worry about ASDs, don't be shy. Screening tests are just that—screening—and don't identify all children with ASDs. The rate of success for the M-CHAT, for example, isn't 100%, so we use it in combination with health and family history to identify children at risk. In my opinion, your opinions as a parent are irreplaceable and of the most importance.

If you are concerned your child has an ASD and your child hasn't been formally screened, talk with your clinician about doing a formal screening. Many screening tools are available for general doctors. But know this: if you are concerned about your child's communication or behavior due to a family history of ASDs, the way he talks or expresses himself, or other people's comments about his behavior, don't wait to talk with the clinician about doing more. If the first doctor doesn't respond to you or take you seriously, get a second opinion.

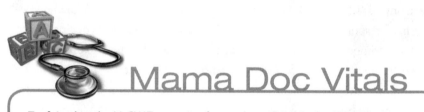

Mama Doc Vitals

Tool: Look at the M-CHAT screening form at http://bit.ly/mdm-MCHAT.

Tip: Early detection is powerful. Autism is a genetic disorder, so no single treatment or medication can cure it. However, early identification and intervention can help children achieve a higher quality of life.

When Not to Worry About Autism Spectrum Disorders

Many parents worry about their child's development at one point or another. With each of my boys, at some point I had worries about their communication and thought their language delays or behaviors signaled something serious. That might just be the worrier in me, but it could just be the mom in me too. Competitive parenting makes us all a little nuts; the act of comparing what our children do against what the cousins or our friends' children do is very difficult to stop. And can make anyone unnerved.

Following are a few signs that your child is developing great communication skills on time. However, if at any time you worry that your child isn't expressing joy, communicating thoughts, or reflecting an understanding of your language, visual cues, and behavior, talk with your child's doctor. If you don't feel heard or you continue to worry, schedule another visit. If you still worry, contact another doctor for a second opinion. Instincts serve us very well when it comes to parenthood. Further, find some peace of mind if your child is doing many of the behaviors listed here!

Reassuring Developmental Milestones for Infants and Children

- Responds to her name between 9 and 12 months of age
- Smiles by 2 months of age; laughs and giggles around 4 to 5 months; expresses great joy to your humor around 6 months
- Plays and thinks peekaboo is funny around 9 months of age
- Makes eye contact with people during infancy
- Tries to say words you say between 12 and 18 months of age
- Uses 5 words by 18 months of age
- Copies your gestures like pointing, clapping, or waving
- Imitates you, ie, pretends to stir a bowl of pancake mix when you give him a spoon and bowl or pretends to talk on the phone with a play cell phone
- Shakes head "no"
- Waves bye-bye by 15 months of age
- Points to show you something interesting or to get your attention by 18 months of age

29

Five Ways to Avoid Cavities

Dental caries (cavities) is preventable for most children. To keep those pearly whites pearly it takes being thoughtful about eating, brushing, and drinking habits and being knowledgeable about your child's water supply. Although physicians are making robots to perform surgery and putting tiny cameras in our bodies to explore the inside, we may sometimes lose sight of easy, affordable ways to improve the lives of millions. Maybe we simply retreat from those prevention efforts…or maybe it's something else.

In 2012, the Centers for Disease Control and Prevention declared for the first time in 40 years that preschoolers had more cavities than they did 5 years prior. And many children have so many cavities that they show up at the dentist with double-digit numbers requiring general anesthesia for repair. In one month alone, I can be asked to do a number of preoperative visits for dental anesthesia for patients in my clinic.

I would suggest there is one thing to stress here. Part of this increase in cavities may be a cultural issue, a parent-culture issue. That is, many parents may not be brushing their children's teeth because of push back from their children and a goal to maintain harmony at home. And many parents believe bottled water is safer than that from the tap. When it comes to teeth, that isn't the case.

Sometimes we really have to act like adults and do the flossing.

I think this bump in cavity numbers is a parenting issue more than anything else. Although factors influencing the development of cavities include access to affordable dentistry, misunderstandings about the safety of fluoride in drinking water, babies going to bed with bottles, and familial risk factors (bacteria in our mouth, for example), we parents clearly play a part too. There are a few things we can do.

Five Tips to Prevent Cavities in Children: The Rule of 2s

1. Take your baby or toddler to the dentist for a checkup before or around her first birthday, even if she only has 2 teeth! The American Academy of Pediatric Dentistry suggests you start checkups no later than 1 year of age (not 3 years). If your dentist sends you away and tells you to return at age 3, find a new dentist.

2. **Use tap water:** Filter it or boil it if you like, but don't buy bottled water for your children. Water with fluoride is protective for your child's teeth. Further, get milk off your baby's or child's teeth prior to bedtime. Never leave a bottle in the crib with your baby, and do your best to brush teeth after her last feed.

3. You heard about Alicia Silverstone's feeding session on YouTube, I assume. The one where she pre-chews her baby's food (pre-mastication) and transfers it back to his mouth? **My advice: don't do this.** You transfer all the cavity-causing bacteria from your mouth to your baby's mouth and increase your baby's risk for early cavities. I feel strongly that parenting like a celebrity isn't always the right way.

4. **Toothpaste!** Use fluoridated toothpaste as soon as your baby gets teeth. You can buy infant toothpaste if you'd like, but it doesn't assist with cleaning better than water. As soon as your baby gets a tooth, use a smear of children's toothpaste (think rice kernel amount) until your child is around 2 years of age and can spit. After they know how to spit, use a pea-sized amount of children's toothpaste.

5. **My rule of 2s:** Brush your child's teeth every day, 2 times a day, until he or she is in second grade, for 2 minutes at a time. Get an egg timer to help because as I learned, that 2 minutes can feel like an eternity with a restless toddler. And if your child wants to try brushing on his own first, fine. But then you clean up the job thereafter.

Flossing every day earns you and your child an A plus. I'm still working on it.

 WendySueSwanson MD @SeattleMamaDoc
Use a tiny (rice kernel amount) of fluoridated toothpaste as soon as your baby/toddler gets teeth. Details: bit.ly/MIFEfg

30

Read the Most Devastating Article

I'm not suggesting this particular article to torture but because it really changed me and my own bias and understanding about forgetfulness, parenting, and risk. "Fatal Distraction" by Gene Weingarten is one of the most devastating articles I've ever read (link in "Mama Doc Vitals" box on page 127).

Parents may leave children in a car that can overheat by accident after forgetting to drop them at school in the morning. As Mr Weingarten writes:

"The wealthy do, it turns out. And the poor, and the middle class. Parents of all ages and ethnicities do it. Mothers are just as likely to do it as fathers. It happens to the chronically absent-minded and to the fanatically organized, to the college-educated and to the marginally literate. In the last 10 years, it has happened to a dentist. A postal clerk. A social worker. A police officer. An accountant. A soldier. A paralegal. An electrician. A Protestant clergyman. A rabbinical student. A nurse. A construction worker. An assistant principal. It happened to a mental health counselor, a college professor and a pizza chef. It happened to a pediatrician. It happened to a rocket scientist."

Children die from hyperthermia after their bodies overheat and exceed 108°F. In 2010, 49 kids died in overheated cars nationwide; then 33 in 2011 and 32 in 2012, according to statistics kept by meteorologist Jan Null and the advocacy group KidsandCars.org. The majority of children who die are younger than 2 years. Infants and toddlers have been forgotten more commonly since the 1990s when experts advised parents to move children to the back seat of cars to prevent injuries from air bags in the front.

Children die after being left in hot cars every year in this country. Typically it's during the summer, of course, but it has happened in 11 different months.

I would suspect you're thinking that you'd never do something like that. You'd never forget your baby…windows up and forgotten, these children die of hyperthermia and overheating. They overheat, cry for help, and are left unheard. It's unthinkable, really.

That's why you must read this article.

Children are particularly vulnerable to heatstroke because their bodies heat up 5 times faster than adults. The reason for their quicker warming stems from children's inferior ability to cool themselves (sweat) and their high surface-area-to-mass ratios.

This utterly alarming trend of children and heatstroke has caught the attention of safety experts. We all need to create systems in our life to prevent this from happening.

Make a system to check the back seat of your car every single time you walk away from it. Kids in it or not.

You can read right over this stuff feeling like it's irrelevant.

You're thinking, this will never happen to me. No way would I forget my kid in the car. Before you convince yourself, read the 2010 Pulitzer Prize–winning article by Gene Weingarten. It has changed my life; it remains one of the most devastating articles I've ever read. I'm not overstating this. The handful of others who I have had read this say the very same. Share it with anyone who will ever drive a child in a car seat or booster seat, anywhere.

What was so staggering about this article was the fact that this could happen to any of us. The problem of children being left in sweltering cars has increased since we have mandated that young children sit in the back seat for safety. The problem of forgetting a child in the car crosses state, racial, socioeconomic, and educational lines.

Parenthood leaves us more and more overwhelmed by life's moment-to-moment tasks. And I'm certainly more forgetful. For example, there have clearly been times when I've

- Left half-empty milk sippy cups in the car for days at a time. We call them "dead milk bottles" for a reason…
- Left the keys to our house hanging in the keyhole in the front door. (Don't get any wise ideas; we've learned our lesson.)
- Left the keys on the roof of the car. Left the wallet at home. Driven to the wrong place.
- Missed a haircut appointment. Plain and simple, got distracted by the day and forgot to go.

These seemingly silly examples of forgetfulness in the overwhelming world of rearing children and working full time illustrate a point. We're all running around at a pace not necessarily ideal for constant thoughtfulness. As the article mentions, stress may really change the way our brain works.

We're all distracted. Not just when we're driving, trying to make dinner, or talking on the phone, but when we're weaving through our simple tasks of daily life. Between my iPhone, e-mail, text messages, patients to see, patients to call back, friend's birthday reminder, alarm to pay the phone bill, early-morning meeting, and the need to remember that Finn likes milk in the green cup and Oden likes milk in the purple, many things are getting forgotten.

God forbid it lead to a devastating mistake.

Five Tips for Anyone With the Privilege of Driving a Child

- *Look before you lock.* Every time you get out of the car, learn to check the back seat. Somehow, make it one of those things you do without thinking. Start today. Walk back to the car if you don't do it the first time you walk away. Make it a rote task like putting on your seat belt.
- Keep your purse, briefcase, or bag in the back seat while driving. A habit that will enforce you checking the back seat and one that will also encourage less use of your phone for texting.
- Share the article by Gene Weingarten with your friends and family. Talking about this story will help affirm its message.
- Don't let children play in a parked car.
- Don't ever hesitate to call 911 if you see a child left unattended in a car.

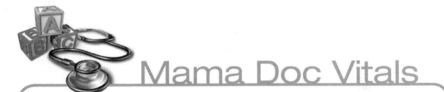

Link: Read the article "Fatal Distraction" by Gene Weingarten at http://bit.ly/mdm-FatalDistraction.

Fact: If it's 80°F outside, your car can heat up to 123°F in an hour. Heatstroke can happen when it's only 60°F to 70°F outside, and we all know from experience that in just 10 minutes, your car can rise 20°F in temperature.

Tip: Have your child's school advised to always call you if your child doesn't show up on a day the school is expecting your child. Build in extra measures of security for protection.

Prepare: Make a 3-Day Disaster Kit

I'm going to be honest: making a disaster kit completely stressed me out. I hope my experience will make it better for you. I'm no expert at this but have learned a lot along the way. And there is no question that I feel so much better with my family prepared and my preparedness tidied.

As *The Economist* stated after Iceland's volcano erupted, "Disasters are about people and planning, not nature's pomp."

So we are left to prepare.

I believe in the 3-tiered approach you see everywhere.

- Make a kit (details to follow).
- Make a plan (how to communicate and find your family).
- Stay informed (what disasters are likely to happen in your area; where to find information).

> *Do your best to buddy up; having a partner was the best move I made.*

I partnered with my friend, Suzan Mazor, MD, who is an emergency department physician. She and I were totally overwhelmed by the task—it just seemed so ominous, even though we knew that it was in our best interest. Do your best to buddy up; having a partner was the best move I made.

The good news: You'll feel better with each step you take and everything you do to prepare your family.

The bad news: This is going to cost you some cash and some time. I spent somewhere between $300 and $350 getting my home and family prepared. And well over 15 hours too.

Double ouch, I know.

First, don't try to reinvent a list. People make these emergency lists for a living and are very good at it. After reviewing multiple Web sites, I really liked the Red Cross list the best for its details for a homemade kit but also its list on communication plans. It's long and overwhelming, but do your best to pick through it.

Pace yourself. You're not going to be able to do this in one day. I'm not entirely done and I've been working on this for a month. You'll need a trip to the grocery store, the hardware store, the bank, the pharmacy, and possibly the doctor's office, then lots of conversations with those in your family so you are all clear about a communication plan. You really want to have a plan to reunite your family in case of an emergency.

After the water, I think the communication plan is what is most important for your family.

Five First Steps for Disaster Planning

1. Go buy two 20-gallon plastic or Rubbermaid-type containers with lids. Once you have those, you'll have a place to organize your emergency gear.

2. Make some *refresh cards*. That is, keep a list on top of your emergency kit of what items need to be replenished and when. I never read about doing this, but with the realities of our busy working-parent-lunatic lives, one of the things we need to do is remind ourselves. Tape an index card to the top of your 20-gallon tub. This is going to be your reminder card for things in the kit that are going to expire. For example, the water I bought expires in 2016; the food, mostly in 2015 but some in 2014. They are on my list. Put a reminder in your cell phone that alarms and reminds you to go to your kit to see your refresh card and replace items.

3. If you can afford a premade family 3-day emergency kit, buy it online today. Then add additional items like clothes for the kids, wrenches, fire extinguishers, medications, and documents. My only complaint about the premade kit we bought is it included water and I really think you can buy that yourself. Furthermore, the water in the kit expired within a year, and the water from the grocery store didn't expire for 2 years. If you can afford the premade kit, it will save you hours.

4. Talk with the other adults in your home and make a plan for where to store your kit, ideally in a garage or lower level near a door. Outside is not a great place to store a kit with food.

5. If your home has natural gas, go and find the area where gas enters your home. Learn how to turn off the gas. Buy a 12-inch Crescent wrench or pliers that allows you to turn it off and leave it at the site of the valve on the outside of your house.

It's OK if you don't finish the following list immediately. I suggest you do this over the next few months. Plan for a few shopping trips—one to the grocery store, one to the computer/Internet, one to the hardware store, and one to the bank.

Grocery Store List

- **Water:** 3 gallons per person or animal. That's a gallon a day for 3 days for every living thing at home. This is the most important thing you have in your kit. You'll need a little more for breastfeeding mothers. Pay attention to expiration dates! It's true that water expires. Just let go of the controversy and believe the experts. If you make your own bottled water, you need to replace those every 6 months.
- **Food:** Buy canned, high-calorie foods that will feed your family for 3 days like chili, tuna, veggies, soup, peanut butter, crackers, and snacks. And some comfort foods like chocolate or candy. Buy foods with similar expiration dates to make it easier to refresh your kit. Don't forget formula for babies and storable milk for toddlers.
- **Medications:** First aid kits don't include these! Specifically, they don't have children's medications. My advice is to include children's or infant acetaminophen (eg, Tylenol) and one container of sunscreen (30 SPF or higher). Also, *write down your infant's or young child's dose of Tylenol* because often the bottle doesn't include it. In a stressed situation, you may forget. Ideally you should have a 7-day supply of any prescription medication you or your child is taking. This is seemingly impractical with the way that insurance companies allow prescription refills (ie, they only give you your month supply). If your child is on an important daily medication, ask your pediatrician for a 1-week supply prescription. Remember to add the expiration date of medications to your refresh card.

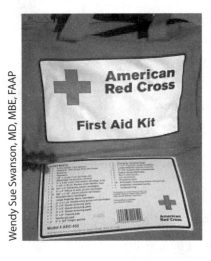

Wendy Sue Swanson, MD, MBE, FAAP

Online Shopping

- **First aid kit:** I recommend buying this online. Kits usually retail for around $25 for a basic kit. Ensure there are a couple pairs of gloves, gauze, tape, and antibiotic ointment.

Hardware Store

- **Tools:** 2 tools stand out as most important to me. One is a wrench for turning off your gas line (if you have it), and two is a can opener. Because, I mean, how peeved would you be if you had your kit, the earthquakes hits, you're chilling with your family, but you couldn't eat the chili. Also, flashlights, batteries, battery- or hand-crank–operated radio, utility knife, waterproof matches, fire extinguisher—one for each floor of your home—nonelectric can opener (as mentioned), and whistles with lanyards for everyone in your home.
- **Sanitation supplies:** Bottle of bleach, hand sanitizer, diapers and wipes, and garbage bags.

> *You'll never be sorry you did this. Promise.*

At-home Tasks

- **Clothing:** A complete change of clothing and shoes for each family member. Hats and gloves. Remember to change this out as your kids grow. Put that on your refresh card!
- **Documents:** Copies of important family documents in a waterproof bag. This one totally stressed me out. Do your best.
- **Entertainment:** Age-appropriate items like a deck of cards, coloring books, or stuffed animals. Maybe old games could live in your kit for a bit?

Overwhelmed? I was too. Hang on, buddy up, and save some money in advance for your kit.

You'll never be sorry you did this. Promise.

Some Good Links

- American Academy of Pediatrics Children & Disasters (www.aap.org/disasters): Resources for health care professionals and families.
- American Red Cross (www.redcross.org): Find information on, for example, lists and communication plans.
- American Red Cross store (www.redcrossstore.org): I went crazy here. I bought a 3-day kit, a hand-crank radio, an emergency escape ladder for our home, and a first aid kit for my car. I didn't expedite shipping and all the goods arrived in fewer than 48 hours. Phew!

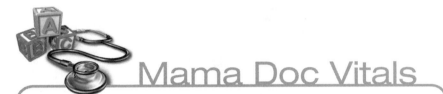

Mama Doc Vitals

Links

- Centers for Disease Control and Prevention Personal Preparation and Storage of Safe Water: http://bit.ly/mdm-SafeWater
- National Resource Center on Advancing Emergency Preparedness for Culturally Diverse Communities 3 Days 3 Ways Disaster Preparedness Workbook: http://bit.ly/mdm-prepare
- Federal Emergency Management Agency Build a Kit: www.ready.gov/build-a-kit

32

What to Do About a Lice Infestation

I really couldn't and wouldn't make this stuff up. We had a lice infestation for the holidays one year. The night before flying out to be with family for Christmas, I was in the midst of typical holiday madness. At one point I was feeling exceedingly proud—I felt for once I'd managed not to get stressed. While in clinic, I made a conscious decision that I wasn't going to stress about the to-do list awaiting me at home. The perspective I get while seeing patients often helps me frame my own stress. Compared to a broken arm or a bout of respiratory syncytial virus (RSV) bronchiolitis, a packing list is really nothing. My husband was on call that night, so when I returned home from clinic around 6:30 pm, the to-do list was mine alone. I needed to pack the family for the holiday, finish off some writing, wrap some gifts, and find something for dinner while completing the holiday cards. I had about 12 hours before we needed to leave for the airport. But this is the life of nearly every parent at one time or another, particularly around the holidays.

Then it hit.

Just before our nanny left, she mentioned that Finn was complaining of an itchy scalp. The rest goes something like this…

Me: "Really? Finn, Lovey, come here, let me look at your head." Pause. Gulp. Wait for it…"You've got to be kidding me; lice for Christmas."

Finn: "Uh-oh."

Finn had lice. Yes, we'd received a letter the week prior that a sibling of one of the preschoolers had lice. The letter seriously sounded like the stories we hear from others about a "friend" with a sexually transmitted infection or a "neighbor's child" who bites. I figured one of the kids in school really did have lice and yes, the threat was there, but then blew it off and went on with life. In 2010, the American Academy of Pediatrics (AAP) put out new recommendations for lice and discouraged schools from sending children home with lice or keeping them away from school. I tend to agree with the recommendations, as having families leave work and sending kids home seems an enormous interruption for a "non-health issue." Maybe because of this, I was just about to have a front-row seat in a major infestation.

Just then, the doorbell rang. *Does this sound like a sitcom?* One of our new neighbors was at the door, huge warm smile on her face. She was inviting us to a quick impromptu holiday party next door. Would I like to come? One of the older children had been offered up to watch the kids so I could head over and have a glass of wine. Pâté. Meet the neighbors, embrace the holidays.

I faked it; I smiled. I don't eat pâté, but a glass of wine sure sounded good. I didn't tell this holiday-cheer–infused welcoming neighbor what was going on. I mean, when someone is standing in your home for the first time, meeting your family and offering pâté and wine, do you tell her your child is covered in bugs?

I shut the door, said I would try to make it (that was the truth), and planned my attack.

First of all, I think (and have previously thought) that lice can be difficult to diagnose. One study found that many presumed "lice" and "nits" submitted by physicians, nurses, teachers, and parents to a laboratory for identification were found to be artifacts such as dandruff, hair spray droplets, scabs, dirt, or other insects (eg, aphids). I'm a pediatrician and I doubted Finn's diagnosis at first. To be honest, I didn't get a lot of training on detecting lice in medical school or residency. It's just simply not a medical issue, so families often don't seek medical care. It may seem easy to find the bugs, but in a restless toddler or preschooler, it can be a feat. Lice also move quickly and avoid the light. Only after I got the über-louse-killing electric-comb thingy at the local pharmacy did I know for certain, in my heart of hearts, that yes, we were dealing with holiday lice.

Most of the statements in pediatric literature and the typical teaching about lice sound something like what the AAP says: "Head lice are not a health hazard or a sign of poor hygiene and, in contrast to body lice, are not responsible for the spread of any disease." It doesn't feel this way as a parent. Nope. Bugs crawling all over your son just doesn't feel devoid of disease. Everything about it, at first, feels hazardous.

Facts help to calm down. Since you started reading this, have you begun to scratch your head?

Head Lice Facts

- Head lice infestation is very common among children 3 to 12 years of age. A 1997 report estimated that approximately 6 to 12 million infestations occur each year in the United States (this may overestimate because the number comes from sales of pediculicides). The AAP says, "Anecdotal reports from the 1990s estimated annual direct and indirect costs totaling $367 million, including remedies and other consumer costs, lost wages, and school system expenses." So a fairly *big* deal, actually.

- Head lice usually survive for less than one day away from the scalp at room temperature. Their eggs cannot hatch at room temperature lower than that near the scalp. So once they fall off a child's head, lice pose very little threat. You don't have to vacuum the carpet, sterilize the toys, or wash the house top to bottom. The August 2010 AAP head lice statement helps clarify: "In 1 study, examination of carpets on 118 classroom floors found no lice despite more than 14000 live lice found on the heads of 466 children using these classrooms. In a second study, live lice were found on only 4% of pillowcases used by infested volunteers." Thus, the AAP suggests that the major focus of control activities should be to reduce the number of lice on the head and to lessen the risks of head-to-head contact.

- With a first case of head lice, itching may not develop for 4 to 6 weeks because it takes that amount of time for sensitivity to result. Lice live near the scalp, feed off blood from little bites, and hatch eggs. The casings of the eggs (nits) are often the easiest thing to see. Nits in some writing refers to the eggs, and in some, just the casings of the eggs.

- Lice are not a hygiene issue. (I'm not just saying this as I out my son, really.) Studies find that contracting lice has nothing to do with bathing standards or socioeconomic level. Translation: anyone, even those with pristine bathing routines and immaculate homes (who are those people?), can get lice!

- Lice spread by crawling (they can't hop or fly). They move from person to person by direct contact. Believe it or not, it's rare for lice to spread via a brush, comb, or shared hat.

Treatment for Head Lice

- **Electric combs:** This is what I started with. I went to my local drugstore and talked with the head pharmacist. The pharmacist recommended the comb. The comb claims to kill lice and eggs (nits) with no toxic exposure. The only precaution on the box was to avoid use in children with epilepsy or pace-makers. At home, within seconds I heard the comb's buzz stop, indicating a dead louse. Within the hour, I had 38 dead lice! I combed and re-combed for more than an hour. After about 20 minutes with no positive results, I stopped my search. Satisfied and exhausted, I thought I had done it. Only issue is that because lice move rapidly and shy away from light, they may be moving about the scalp while you work. This made me a little crazy. I kept combing and re-combing and re-combing…and the result? On re-combing the following day (now in California with the in-laws), I found 2 more live lice! That's when I decided to go for a pediculicide. Santa was on his way, and I felt I had no choice. Bottom line: I think these combs can work well but not 100% of the time. They are tedious, and you'll never know for certain each bug or egg is killed because lice can move during treatment. If you choose to use one, you'll need to repeat your work daily for 7 to 14 days—a *huge* time commitment. I couldn't find any good research studies and data on these combs. Further, the AAP states, "No randomized, case-controlled studies have been performed with either type of comb."
- **Pediculicides:** These are chemical treatments that kill lice and eggs/nits. One-percent permethrin lotion (eg, Nix) is currently recommended as one of the drugs of choice for head lice in the United States. It claims to kill lice and their eggs for 14 days. However, because of silicon-based additives in most shampoos/conditioners that remain on the hair shaft, there is concern that the permethrin may not stick to the shaft of the hair well and allow for ongoing killing of eggs. Many experts recommend re-treatment at 7 days and then again at 13 to 15 days after the first dose.
- **Hot air:** A 2006 study in *Pediatrics* found that using hot dryers called LouseBusters (now called AirAllé) for 30 minutes (think salon-type hair-dryer chairs) may be a great cure for lice. In the study, the 30-minute treatment was found to kill 88% to 100% of the lice (depending on which brand of dryer). I can't recommend against them, but they may be difficult to find in your area. Until they are found more readily, it's hard to know how effective and useful they are.

- **Benzyl alcohol:** The US Food and Drug Administration approved use of 5% benzyl alcohol in 2009. The product is not neurotoxic and kills head lice by asphyxiation (suffocation). Studies demonstrated that more than 75% of the subjects treated were free of lice 14 days after initial treatment. Not perfect, but not bad. It doesn't kill the eggs so you have to retreat at 7 and maybe 13 to 15 days, even if you're a master with the nit comb. You need a prescription for this.

- **Lindane:** I don't recommend it because it is considered neurotoxic and there have been numerous reports of seizures after use. With all the other options out there, avoid it. I'd say it's better to have bugs.

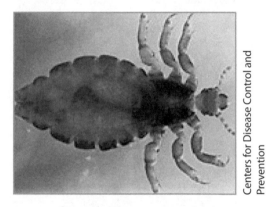

Centers for Disease Control and Prevention

So What About Nit Picking?

Until now, I'd never understood the rationale for nit picking when pediculicides kill live lice and eggs/nits. You may not need to do the combing, but your freedom from the comb will depend on your decision to re-treat. Reality is, none of the pediculicides are perfectly 100% ovicidal (egg-killing). So removal of nits (especially the ones within 1 cm of the scalp) after treatment with any product is recommended. Nit removal can be tedious and challenging (I'LL SAY!). However, combing every last centimeter of your child's hair may be worth your while. The AAP states that studies have suggested that lice removed by combing and brushing are damaged and rarely survive. So at least you'll add to your electric comb, permethrin (Nix), or benzyl alcohol efforts.

Many urban areas have hair salons and private business that specialize in removing lice—and most offer a guarantee. If you're not up for the lice-zapping electric comb or permethrin shampoos and subsequent nit picking, you can hire this out. I've known other friends who have done this and were satisfied.

I'll admit that when we had lice infestation number 2, we chose to do this and were very satisfied.

Although the whole experience of using an electric comb followed by drowning our heads of hair in permethrin one day later wasn't ideal, it did feel a bit like a rite of passage in parenting. In the end, lice didn't feel like disease, just incredibly disgusting and disruptive.

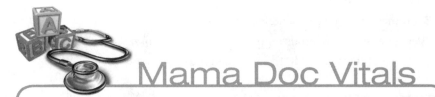

Mama Doc Vitals

Tip: The most important thing you do when your child has lice is nit pick and comprehensively comb. Then repeat daily for 7 to 14 days.

Facts: Head lice cannot hop or fly. To spread, they have to crawl from one person to another. Pets do not play a role in lice infestations. Not fair to blame the dog!

Part 2

Social-Emotional Support

SOCIAL-EMOTIONAL GROWTH

We all want our children to grow up into healthy, happy, and positive people. But how do we help them do this? Follow these simple ways to help your child get a healthy dose of character growth every day.

GRATITUDE

Best Part of Day (BPOD)
Each day, have everyone in the family say what their best part of the day was.

ESTEEM

Teasing Out Self-talk
Let your children know that self-talk (your inner voice) exists, and help them balance stressful thoughts with positive ones.

GENEROSITY

Inspire Generosity
Help children give to others both in full view (donating to a school food drive) and in priva* (dropping off gifts anonymously).

RESPONSIBILITY

The Saturday Box
The Saturday Box claims anything that's been lying out for a while (parents' things too!); what gets claimed is gone until Saturday. This gives kids a sense of communal responsibility in their own micro-community.

SELF-REGULATION

Learning to Lose
A competitive spirit is great, but remind kids that everyone is in it to win—sometimes it's just not "in the cards."

Surviving Tantrums
During a tantrum, offer small choices with directed options (not yes/no)—having a little control can help calm children down.

Separation Anxiety
Practice being apart, whether it's off to Grandma's or preparing for first-day-of-school good-byes. Prepare your children to thrive in your absence!

PLAY

Be Without a Ceiling
Go outside with your children every day. Move in a space that has no ceiling. Weather is no excuse!

Just Play
Provide opportunities each day for your children to just play. Let them delight in the freedom to create, imagine, and associate with others.

Unplugging
Take a restorative 24 hours off-line from sundown Friday to sundown Saturday. No phones, tablets, or computers!

MINDFULNESS

Mindful Parenting
Mindfulness (the art of non-doing) is an opportunity to grow into precious moments alone and then alongside our children.

f you follow the right path, helping our children grow emotionally and ocially is fun, impactful, and the est part of each day for you and our children.

Part 2
Social-Emotional Support

Introduction

The Seattle Mama Doc blog and the writing here has catered to one principle I've learned along the way in life: *Parents just want to do what is right.* The desperate love we have for our children can shock us into good and sometimes bad decisions. I believe parents search for and sincerely desire simple answers to how-what-why-who, the essence of doing right for their children. Often it's not a simple, isolated situation or as complicated as it may feel. And the abundance of online noise invokes fear in all of us. In writing, I want to illuminate the reality that in pediatrics, doing less is often more. Prevention reigns.

Parents just want to do what is right.

It's defining what's *right* that on occasion remains elusive.

We all want information to facilitate decisions that let us rest easier at night. Having my own 2 children makes this reach for what is right palpable. It's a very real challenge to juggle the demands of daily life with that of helping support thoughtful, insightful, consistent, sound advice for our children. In in my life as a pediatrician and mother, I've found I have to look to others and to stories and the wisdom of the crowd to help me raise my boys intelligently. I really want them to have big margins to be who they are but to also respect those around them.

I will share my stories and tell how it all feels to me. I ask my colleagues, peers, and friends for help and uncover powerful lessons to share; some are captured here. I do my best to offer helpful online resources and share methods I learn from patients, friends, and family, in and out of medicine, to help me find answers. The hope, of course, is to support our children's social-emotional learning and growth and to remember that it's easier than we thought, not elusive after all.

33

BPOD: Best Part of Day

Make gratitude a daily part of your children's lives. The trick is to embed easy habits that take little time; that way, research shows, the habits stick. Ease is essential for lasting permanence. We love one new tradition and it's adding to our well-being. Being mindful of what we have in our lives—people, experiences, opportunities—has remarkable power.

We started a new tradition in 2012. We started going around the table every single night announcing our BPOD, our *Best Part of Day*. What's been so amazing about it is that we've been doing it every single day with anyone who joins us for dinner and any family members who are around. In the beginning, Finn and Oden, 3 and 5 years old at the time, kind of imitated each other. They started out by saying the same thing; if we were outside flying a kite, I knew it was coming. I knew at the end of the day they'd announce it was their BPOD.

But now, something's really changed in our house. Now that we've been doing it for more than a year, our children are thinking about their days differently. I know when something's happening that's really exciting during the day. Their codifying it, putting it in their library, and even in the middle of the day, my son will reach over and say, "Hey! This is my BPOD."

Mindful of something wonderful, they seemed to be witnessing gratitude in the moment.

Sometimes the announced BPOD stays all the way until dinner, and sometimes it doesn't. It's been a magical and wonderful transition. We're all looking forward to dinner in a different way, and every time we sit down, one of our kids often reminds us it's time for BPOD.

Think about starting a BPOD in your house. A tradition to share the best part of your day, every day. And call it a BPOD so it sticks. Gratitude is powerful stuff.

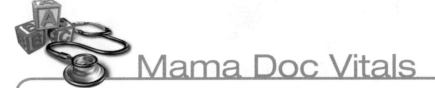

Mama Doc Vitals

Tip: Get in the habit of doing a BPOD every day. After a week or so you won't have to be in charge—your children will remind you!

Fact: Practicing gratitude can increase happiness. Significant psychological research suggests that happiness is related to being grateful for what we already have.

Video: Watch this video, in which I talk about BPOD: http://bit.ly/mdm-BPODvideo.

34

Helping Your Anxious Child: Blowing Colors

Anxiety and anxious feelings are a normal part of every childhood. However, some children really do get amped up in different ways. Often we see children's stress and anxious feelings come out at times of transitions or at bedtime. Some children really do have a hard time winding down at night. It's not always anxiety, but it can disrupt sleep.

This is a little trick I use to help coach anxious children whose minds just seem to "spin." Patients have given me great feedback over the years that *blowing colors* really helps. Sometimes it's for children and teens who can't drift off to sleep, sometimes for those who are worriers, and sometimes for those who get anxious or overwhelmed at school. Blowing colors is a great exercise to return to regular belly-breathing patterns, buy time and space for mindfulness, and improve control over feelings of being overwhelmed. See if it helps.

Greatest thing is—this is a good tool for a child or teen to regain control. He can use the exercise anywhere, at any time. Lots of children and teens who get anxious feel ashamed of their anxiety and don't want to reach out for help. Reassure them that no one will ever know they're blowing colors or changing the hue of a room. Practice at home before bed or in school during moments of being overwhelmed, or even remind a child or teen that he can blow colors while out with friends or at a sleepover.

When you're anxious and nervous, you breathe just from your chest, short little breaths. We can learn from babies who do belly breathing, those deep breaths where your diaphragm moves up and down. We know that can increase blood flow and hopefully calm kids down.

Teach Children to Blow Colors

- Outline and spell out the 3-dimensional room that you are in and talk to your child about all the air in that space.
- Talk to her about how you can see your breath in the wintertime when it's really cold out. Establish the reality that each time you breathe you move volumes of air.
- Then imagine each and every big puff of breath that your child makes is in a different color. Teach her to take those big breaths and blow a color.

- Tell your child to imagine filling the entire room with puffs of orange, yellow, or green.

Some kids will even say that as they start to turn a room blue or purple, they really start to relax and sometimes even drift off to sleep....

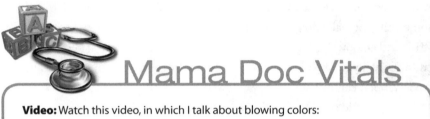

Video: Watch this video, in which I talk about blowing colors: http://bit.ly/mdm-BlowingColors.

Children With Gay Parents

Headlines like "Children Do Better With Committed Parents" excite me. I feel proud to live in a time where we're advancing understanding and safety for children and their health—I love being a part of it. Over the past decade(s) there have been big shifts here in the United States. In mid-2013, the Pew Research Center published data demonstrating that there has been a notable change in public opinion when it comes to the nation's support of gay marriage; more people support gay marriage (50%) than oppose it (43%). In particular, 66% of millennials (people aged 18–32 years) support gay marriage.

Earlier in 2013, the American Academy of Pediatrics (AAP) stepped forward in support of gay marriage in hopes of improving child well-being nationwide. The AAP, a group that represents 60,000 pediatricians who care for families all over the United States, did so not for politics but for children.

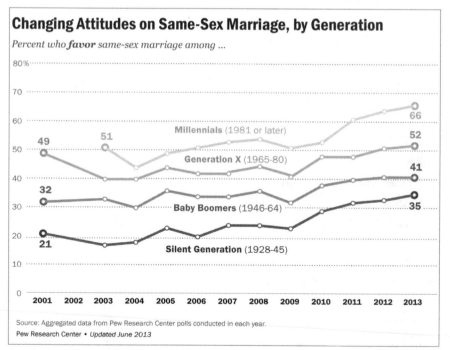

Changing Attitudes on Same-Sex Marriage, by Generation

Percent who favor same-sex marriage among ...

Millennials (1981 or later) — 49, 51, ... 66
Generation X (1965-80) — 52
Baby Boomers (1946-64) — 41
Silent Generation (1928-45) — 32, ... 35, 21

Source: Aggregated data from Pew Research Center polls conducted in each year.
Pew Research Center • Updated June 2013

Pew Research Center, "Changing Attitudes on Same-Sex Marriage, by Generation," June 6, 2013, http://features.pewforum.org/same-sex-marriage-attitudes/index.php. Reprinted with permission.

There are mounting piles of research that the estimated 2 million children being raised by gay or lesbian parents are doing beautifully. In fact, the AAP says, "…more than 100 scientific publications over 30 years, taken together, have demonstrated that children's well-being is affected much more by their relationships with their parents, their parents' sense of competence and security, and the presence of social and economic support for the family than by the gender or the sexual orientation of their parents."

The statement shed more insight into the beautiful, healthy lives children lead when in a supportive, loving home. There aren't data to suggest that heterosexual couples raise healthier children.

Federal support of gay marriage was historically finicky. The federal Defense of Marriage Act (DOMA) previously deprived children of gay parents (even those living in the 13 states plus Washington, DC, that allow gay marriage) access to federal rights and benefits other children of married parents receive—things like social security, housing and food stamps, employment benefits, military benefits, and even taking child deductions on jointly filed federal taxes. Therefore, for the well-being of families and children everywhere, the AAP supported the position that DOMA was unconstitutional and should be repealed.

Fortunately, in June 2013, the US Supreme Court ruled that DOMA was unconstitutional. Therefore, the restrictions in access to resources were taken away for children with gay parents. The repeal was a huge step toward ensuring that children everywhere have increased protection.

In the AAP policy statement and accompanying technical report (which reviews data more extensively), the organization says, "…laws restricting competent adults of the same gender from codifying their commitment to each other and their children via civil marriage may result not only in pain and hardship for their children but also in legal, economic, psychological, social, and health disparities that can no longer be justified."

I stand behind the AAP in its move to support children in all diverse family units. Providing structure, security, financial benefits, health benefits, and access to federal programs equally has to be what we do for children in our nation. Children and families thrive with structure. Because only 13 states (plus Washington, DC) in the United States allow for same-sex marriage and many states don't forbid discrimination of adoptive and foster-care parents who are gay and lesbian, repealing DOMA was essential to ensuring that all children have the same rights to security around our nation.

I see it like this: stability is good for children. Things like having meals with your family, having access to a safe school and quality health care, and even living in a home that requires a regular bedtime help. Stability in rights and resources because of marriage matters to children too. Children are and will always be dependent on their parents in part for stability. Getting rid of DOMA restrictions demonstrated progress for all of our children.

36

Love: Unequal and Incomparable

When I was pregnant with my second son, I had no idea how much I would love him. It didn't seem possible that I could love him like I did my first. As I awaited his arrival (on bed rest), my expectations for him grew, but my projected love and feelings remained very measured. I imagined having a blueprint for love, a near duplicate map of that with my first son. I was imagining a replica; I had no other schema for having a baby of my own. In this space, I expected it would all feel very familiar in my heart. And although this hope and anticipation fueled my pregnancy, I remember housing doubt that I would have the capacity to love another like I loved my first son. In some moments, it didn't seem possible; the love already felt immense and unconstrained. As any parent knows, it's simply insurmountable to quantify or govern love for your child.

If anything, I think I expected my love to feel equal for each boy, despite not understanding the mechanics of how it would happen. Part of that came from my mother telling me that she loved my brother and me equally when we were growing up. This often came up at incredibly sentimental times (note: sarcasm) like epic battles in sharing or when choosing which one of us needed to take the garbage out.

Of course, I'm sure my mom's feelings are more complex, but her assertion of equality was the foundation in my thinking.

Out popped Oden in 2008. And just like everyone said, I fell in love with him…desperately.

But my love wasn't simple; it wasn't the same. My heart didn't mimic any pattern I'd developed for Finn. Oden was an entirely unique person in my life. And I generated an entirely new sense of connection.

My love for my boys isn't "equal" in height, weight, or circumference. The love I feel for Oden is absolutely incomparable to the love I feel for Finn. As if it's a different color, a different language, a different texture, or a different tonality. The space they occupy in me is immense and limitless, separate, and only occasionally overlapping. I don't love one more than the other, but I can't articulate how I love them in unequal ways. But I do.

Does the love you feel for your child equal that for anything else?

WendySueSwanson MD @SeattleMamaDoc

Today my son F said, "I just love you, Mommy." It was the "just" that went straight to my heart. #parenting

---

Mindful Parenting

There was a moment just after President Obama was sworn into office in January 2013 that I'd seen on TV that I returned to in my thoughts relentlessly. The President turned amid the regal archway of the Capitol and stopped. His accompanying family and tribe of lawmakers waited. The myriad of microphones picked up that he said something like, "I want to take a look one more time." And then he looked back on the National Mall and seemed to take it all in. A few seconds, maybe half a minute or so. Not long, no, but the moment seemed to take up enormous space. Quietly, eyes wide open, he looked out to the millions who had come to celebrate and bear witness to his honor and his responsibility. Instead of looking at him, my eyes migrated to his daughter, Malia. I saw her watching.

It may have been mindfulness she saw.

It's of course never clear to an outsider who is mindful or not. Thinking and spending energy to be more present is a pastime that I was introduced to as a medical student because of the work of Jon Kabat-Zinn, PhD. I use lessons from his work in my personal and professional life on a daily basis. Therefore, it was a sincere joy to sit amid 1,000 other parents and hear Dr Kabat-Zinn and his wife Myla talk about *mindful parenting*. I was surrounded by my husband and friends, many colleagues and pediatricians, and I was lucky enough to sit near parents of my patients. It was community. To me it felt like a needed touchstone and a hearty reminder of how nicely being mindful fits into a busy, reflective, hectic, and imperfect life.

The following day I had the privilege of also having lunch with the Kabat-Zinns and a group of psychologists and pediatricians to sit and discuss mindfulness in pediatrics. Chewy, good things.

Five Lessons From the Kabat-Zinns on Mindful Parenting

- Mindfulness is not the antithesis of anything. There is no single ill or evil that impedes it. In fact, the last question on the night from the audience begged the Kabat-Zinns to detail the biggest obstacle to mindfulness. They couldn't answer it, really. All this precisely because mindfulness in its simplicity is openness, compassion, and love. At the opening of the talk, Jon helped us recognize the work that it took to bring us there, amid the heavy Thursday raindrops, rush hour traffic, busy workweeks, needy toddlers or teens at home, and the truth that there was potentially something else we really should be doing. He reminded us all that it was LOVE that had brought us together to listen to ideas about mindful parenting. This we all share. This is why mindfulness is possible for everyone at every time in their life. Each new moment is evolving into something entirely new.

- At one point, Dr Kabat-Zinn looked down at his watch. At first glance it appeared he was tracking the timing of his talk, and then he burst out, "If you check your watch, it's now again." A hilarious reminder that each and every moment that unfolds is always now. We have a chance to bear witness to time indefinitely. We are offered up the opportunity to be mindful, open, and present with an infinite number of do-overs. Oh, wow—it's now again. Myla furthered this, saying, "Every moment is the possibility of a new beginning." Every single moment is a new chance to be aware.

- Parenting is overwhelming governed by love. Being mindful, ever present, and always full of love is an impossibility. Suffering is a part of being human, whether you're an adult or child, they reminded. But the potential for seeing the world alongside our children, with the backdrop of the sky, is always there. Kabat-Zinn refreshingly stated that we had "live-in teachers" for mindfulness because of our children. Think of the moments each child takes and absorbs in her days. And think how often she ushers you into the world differently. Parenting is a privilege, and having these teachers around us is true wealth, but it's not necessarily easy. Our children will teach us about mindfulness naturally, but we'll likely be startled to learn that we think the curriculum is one thing while they repeatedly demonstrate it's something altogether different. Think of it—just when you think you've planned the perfect mindful afternoon for a picnic with your child, her experience of it will turn into something new—an afternoon hunt for a lost ball or day to ask for crackers. These teachers really will surprise us.

- Mindfulness is the art of non-doing. There is nothing prescriptive about it—no real how-to bullet points to share. Rather, be reminded that our society will not feature this—it isn't sexy or exciting or easy to market, not being productive. Not doing, stretching into a moment's enormity, is a way to grow into ourselves. And this will serve our children, not only ourselves. When we model mindfulness, not just attempt to enter the moment our children observe, but when we find our own moment, we may be the most helpful. Think of President Obama. Think of his keen daughter watching as he stopped his gait, turned on his heel, and looked out to the people who elected him to lead. Think of the power we have when we take in, stop judging, and open ourselves up to a moment. Our children, at every age, are watching.

- The Kabat-Zinns reminded us that we can have anger for anyone. Stop being alone in that. Someone 40 days old and someone 40 months or 40 years old has the potential to infuriate us. This is steeped in our love. Size and age are irrelevant when it comes to inciting fire. "We save our ire for those we care about the most," they said. This acknowledgment is essential in parenting. Feeling anger, frustration, deep disappointment, and fire in your heart for those you love the most is human. It may not be forgiveness that we need but space to see and feel the anger and then find our own way out. Each and every moment will pass and evolve into another.

WendySueSwanson MD @SeattleMamaDoc

"Someone 40 days old & someone 40 months or 40 years has the potential to infuriate us." On Mindful Parenting: bit.ly/10K2HmP

Mindfulness isn't just about a loss of distraction. It isn't as easy as those blog posts from moms who are reborn into a new world without their cell phone. Mindfulness is at its essence far more simple yet far more complex than that. It's the opportunity we have to grow into the precious moment we are given again and again—uniquely, alone, and then entirely alongside our children with the backdrop of the sky. Each day a chance again.

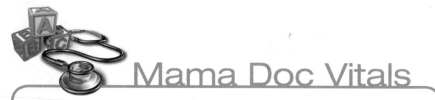

Mama Doc Vitals

Books: For more on the Kabat-Zinns' lessons, check out their books *Everyday Blessings* and *Full Catastrophe Living*.

38

Teasing Out Self-talk: Our Inner Critic

Soon after my oldest son started kindergarten, I had the good fortune to hear Jim Webb, PhD, give a lecture on the emotional needs of children.

During his talk he mentioned children and their self-talk. *Self-talk* is that voice that constantly evaluates how you're doing things, how the world is playing out, and ultimately how you feel about it. That voice that tells us to hurry up, berates us when we feel we've messed up, and often wakes us up in a moment of daydreaming to get us back on track.

Most of us have a lot of negative self-talk. And it starts early in childhood.

Dr Webb, a psychologist, shared the tip that we can tease out the inner critic our children have too. Not only can we mention that this self-talk exists, we can demonstrate and model that voice for our children. We can show them we also have a voice that hovers to illuminate what we do wrong or what we do well.

We can make light that this voice is always here. We can tame it too. My self-talk is more a critic than a coach.

Dr Webb made me realize that we identify this self-talk early and help children acknowledge and own it. If I remember correctly, no one taught me about my self-talk growing up. I wonder if they had if my critic would be a bit more forgiving or generous…. Maybe we can help our children identify their inner critic and help them shape their critic into a more productive coach. Just knowing self-talk exists and bearing witness to this critic could be a great start to insight.

Teach Children About Self-talk Early

- Teach children that self-talk exists. Once children are in school, start mentioning and letting them know that their voice and inner critic is there. Help them recognize the self-talk they are participating in and ask them how it helps them during the day. Ask them if it trips them up.
- Teach children about the errors we make in self-talk. Think about the tone of your own critic—what proportion of the day is your self-talk positive versus negative? Think about the proportion of the day as if it's a pie chart. If you're like most people, your self-talk is often predominately negative.

- Talk about what Dr Webb calls "the bookkeeping errors" we make. Help your children learn to keep better books. Think about how it often seems that the mistakes or misspeaks of our day tend to overrule the triumphs or contributions we make. Self-talk, particularly with those children prone to perfectionism, can contribute to anxious or depressed feelings. It's true that society proves this to us again and again—one lie can undo 10,000 truths in a political career, for example. But when it comes to our inner critic, we may be able to shape a more perfect union. Talk to your children about how their critic can keep more accurate books.

Model your own self-talk—including when it goes south on you (when appropriate)—and work together with your children to acknowledge it's there.

Self-talk is a very private event and always will be. But one thing we can likely give our children is a better way to grow into themselves…coach or critic included.

39

New Rule: Be Without a Ceiling

I've got a new rule. And this is coming from a woman who grew up in Minnesota and who lives in Seattle. I'm stating clearly first: weather is no excuse.

I've talked in many places about the reality that there are only a few "rights" to parenting. In my opinion, as a mom and pediatrician, the rare "rights" or "corrects" of parenthood include things like getting your children immunized and properly using car and booster seats. Beyond that, the rest of parenting is a smattering of "doing right," versions that vary and resonate from person to person and child to child. The thing is, most of us do it very well, without strict rules. That is, out of love and instinct, we parent our children beautifully and get them to adulthood intact and insightful. We shelter them. Protect them. Feed them. Shield them from harm. Provide opportunity.

Often, the information we read about parenting does more to break our spirits than it does to bolster phenomenal, inventive ideas. And even though a physician friend recently told me that he subscribes to "good-enough" parenting, and that I tend to agree, I believe this week I've stumbled on the third possible "right" (versus a "wrong"). Please write me, tweet me, and tell me if you think I'm wrong because I just can't conceptualize the counterargument to my claim and new rule.

> Go outside with your children every day. Move in a space that has no ceiling.

With the rising digital demand on our lives and technology seeping into every space, getting outside remains one basic and beautiful way to stay healthy, connected, and opportunistic with your children. And better yet, it's a great way for your children to be afforded the luxury to roam, create, and play. Not only will your children move and exercise, they'll experience nature. Nature, as simple as the sticks on the sidewalk or the grass in the boulevard, or nature, like the spaces where you see, hear, smell, touch nothing man-made. All of it, any of it, every day. It seems to me that nature is something we've nearly forgotten to prioritize with our time here on Earth.

Even if outside time is only 15 minutes, prioritize being outside in your life with your children.

So don the coat, mittens, hat, or sunscreen. Whenever illness doesn't get in your way, do whatever you can to remain comfortable and protected, then get outside each and every day with your children.

Move in a space with no ceiling.

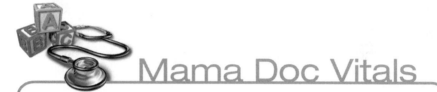

Mama Doc Vitals

Tip: Get one-way tickets on the bus or let your spouse or partner drop you and your children off to a dinner out or a friend's house. Plan to walk home after dinner or a playdate—even in the rain!

Fact: Childhood obesity has more than doubled for adolescents and more than tripled for children in the last 30 years. This is in part due to increasing levels of inactivity…

Fact: Nature-deficit disorder was coined by Richard Louv in his 2005 book *Last Child in the Woods.* Louv believes people, especially children, are spending less time outdoors, resulting in a wide range of behavioral problems.

40

Learning to Lose?

We spent a fair bit of one of our weeks of vacation when the boys were 3 and 5 years old playing 2 games, Uno and Spot It. At the time, our son Finn was acting wholly competitive; he likes to know all the answers, and he likes to win. He really likes to play and at the time giggled when things would go his way or when throwing a "Skip" or "Draw 4" card in Uno. But he also began to show us how much he hates to lose. It turns out he's rarely wrong about things, so not having things go his way isn't really a part of his evolving schema. Thing is, he is also really polite. So when his behavior disappoints us, he takes things seriously. He hates it when we're disappointed.

After losing at both Uno and Spot It one Thursday afternoon, he began collapsing in the chair, throwing his excess remaining (losing) cards onto the table (or the floor) in frustration and sighing. After a second dramatic display, I'd had it. I told him he must sit out a game the next time we all got to play. I used the rationale, "Your friends won't want to play games with you if you can't celebrate when they win." And, "Everyone playing the game is aiming for the same goal; we all want to win. Sometimes it just won't be in the 'cards' for you."

I told him he simply must be polite and celebrate others when they win.

The next game he got to play was Uno, and his grandmother won. Just when she did he said, "Congratulations, Grandma. Well done." He held onto his cards. He smiled. It was verbatim to how I'd instructed him. There was a plastered smile on his face. Something wasn't quite right. And I must admit, something about it didn't seem desirable. Without authenticity, I wasn't so sure I was doing it right.

About 2 hours after the game, my husband Jonathan read a passage aloud to me from *The New Yorker* about Peter Thiel and his desire to win, stemming back to his math prowess as a child and his inclination for chess.

Peter Thiel became a math prodigy and a nationally ranked chess player. He later became a very successful entrepreneur and investor (he cofounded PayPal and was the original investor in Facebook). So something about him really understands strategies for winning and success.

The New Yorker article described how Thiel's chess kit was decorated with a sticker carrying the motto, "Born to Win." Apparently, on the rare occasions when he lost in college, he was known to act a bit like a tyrant and sweep the pieces off the board. After his adolescent tantrums, he would say, "Show me a good loser, and I'll show you a loser."

And there you are. This man, once a ruthless childhood winner, grew up to be a remarkably successful person. I'm left wondering, how good a loser should we all be? What part fighting-spirit-competitor is necessary to allow our children to reach their potential and contribute in big ways? Something about that moment where Finn exclaimed the rote, "Congratulations, Grandma," just didn't seem right. Polite, yes. Being respectful is requisite in my mind and necessary for most of us for living a connected, compassionate, and productive life. But the inauthentic first try at "Congratulations, Grandma," left me in a parenting perplexity. The question really is, do you want to create an obstinate-genius-winner or a good loser? I must admit, part of me really doesn't know. But I'm certain there is something in between…

41

Plan a Vacation, *Stat*

As Memorial Day weekend slips into the rearview mirror each spring, we set our sights on summertime. Often that includes a camping trip or vacation away from home. When it comes to travel, there are data supporting how to do summertime *right*. The short version: plan a vacation today. Stop whatever you're doing, take a marker to the calendar, and block off some time for your family. Trust me, it may make you happy. Right now.

Being happy, chasing happy, and achieving/experiencing happiness are often motivators (or excuses) for the decisions we make. Despite the ubiquitous quest for happiness and the countless books we can read, it eludes many of us. When reading about happiness, we often hear about *mindfulness,* the focus on the present and doing our best to live in the moment in which we live.

For happiness, we often hear about regaining simplicity.

It seems that if we just stopped planning and thinking about the future or worrying with regret about the past, we'd find ourselves entirely aware and entirely much happier. When it comes to summer vacations, data are different.

A 2010 Dutch study found that planning for the vacation, not the vacation itself, makes you happy. We really must focus on anticipation (vacation planning) if we're going to get the best out of our trips and travels! Positive effects of vacations don't last long. Previous work finds that those of us who suffer from burnout return to our pre-vacation levels of stress and being overwhelmed just 3 to 4 weeks after vacation ends. Therefore, the Dutch study can guide us in really making the most of our limited time away.

- Researchers surveyed 1,530 people about their vacation planning, length of stay, holiday stress, frequency of travel, health status, and personality type (extroversion). They used happiness scales. They sought to determine which part of a vacation really makes us happy.
- Pre-trip happiness was notably different between groups, while post-trip happiness was not. There was a statistically significant difference between vacationers versus those staying home prior to the trip. However, after the trip, the significant differences in happiness scores between the groups faded away.

- Data from the study support the notion that multiple short trips in a summer (or year) provide more happiness than one long trip because of the pre-trip anticipation boost of happiness. Vacations that lasted 2 weeks seemed to provide "very relaxed" trips more often than short ones, although in general, the effects of longer vacations don't tend to persist or differ once we return to work. As we all know, the e-mail inbox can overwhelm us once we return no matter how long we're away.

Note to self: planning for a long weekend (or many long-weekend journeys) may make you just as happy as planning for a 2-week trip to the beach.

People derive more happiness from 2 or more short breaks spread throughout the year than from having just a single longer holiday once a year.

So this really is about the moment—the moment before the trip. Although travel with our children is rigorous (I like to call travel with infants and toddlers "trips," not "vacation"), the goal isn't only happiness, of course. Travel with children is about memories, explorations, wandering, protected family time, and cultural exposure too.

Planning the trip turns out to be an exquisitely important part.

Go get that permanent marker; block off some time. To boost our levels of delight, it makes sense to plan far in advance with our children. Start a countdown today. We'll get more and more out of that pre-trip mood boost the more lead time we have. Even if only a single-day trip, the anticipation may really pay off.

42

Why the Pony Doesn't Win

I was reminded why the pony doesn't win. When I was finished with bedtime stories, I sat on the edge of Finn's bed. He was nearing 4½ years old (he counted the days) and was full of ideas but also still busting with thoughtfulness. We'd had a day out of a storybook. Really. It started with an Easter party (with chocolate!) at a neighbor's home, an Easter egg hunt at our local park, a spotting of *the* Easter Bunny, a balloon artist, and A PONY RIDE. A pony ride! By the end of the day, the sun was out and I was full, satiated, calm, and feeling very connected to my boys. Jonathan was on call at the hospital, so I had the boys primarily to myself for the majority of the day. As we readied for a night of sleep, we snuggled in. Mindful of the day and noting the space, I finished reading the book and asked him a question. I wouldn't have thought to tell you the next part, but you'll need to know more to understand his answer.

After the hoopla of the morning, my mom came over. The clouds opened and the sun joined us. When Finn didn't take a nap, I invited him outside to help my mom and me dig holes, haul dirt, and put new plants in the ground. The sun was warm and evident; the dirt wasn't wet. The hand trowel, just Finn's size. He helped us prepare the new plants, move small rocks out of the way, and put peat and soft fluffy soil around the newly potted plants. He was an integral part of our landscaping team. We were thankful. His enthusiasm ushered me through hours of yard work (not usually my favorite task).

"What was your favorite part of the day?" I asked just before I left the room and turned out the light.

A beat went by. It was as if he was going through the Rolodex of the day.

"Gardening," he said matter-of-factly.

See? Life is really about who you're with and how you fit in amid your people. It's this connection, this sense of contribution, this sense of completion that can keep us going. Part of why it's often just so nice to help. Even a pony doesn't overpower how good it can be to feel included and useful. See? The pony doesn't always win.

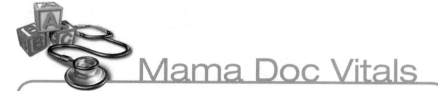

Mama Doc Vitals

Tip: When you plan a perfect day and things go miserably, remember that magical ones will appear when you least expect it. Perhaps even when your child refuses to nap one day.

Link: Try this → Design a beautiful day: http://bit.ly/mdm-BeautifulDay.

Fact: Most children stop napping around ages 4 to 5 years. Some children stop napping as early as 18 months of age, but 25% of 5-year-olds still nap. That's a big range of normal.

43

Anything for a Nap

So you know that thing you do when you're desperate for your kid to sleep? That thing where you take your child to the park, run him into the ground, and force him to stay up a bit later than usual? Then when nearing complete destruction or implosion, you keep the windows down in the car and the music blaring so he won't fall asleep on the way home? All this in the hopes that when you are home, he CRASHES. CRASHES HARD and sleeps like a zombie. Instinct tells you that the physical fatigue your child acquires will allow him to pound out an outrageous nap.

We do this. Most of us, at least. I did this. We think that the way we sleep is the same as the way our kids sleep. And after learning by experience that a hard day of weeding, running, or traveling increases our ability to crash asleep, we trust that tiring out our kids will get them to nap extra-hard, extra-soundly, and extra-long.

Brutal reality: it may not, at least not all the time.

One rare example when our instincts may not serve us well. Especially if your child isn't a pro sleeper to begin with. Children have different sleep needs, of course, and different sleep patterns than adults.

One of my friends and colleagues, Maida Chen, MD, FAAP, helped me understand this more clearly. She's a pediatric pulmonologist and sleep specialist. She's the bomb—a mom, a lung doctor, a sleep doctor, a wife to a radiologist, and a practical clinician. She knows a ton about understanding sleep and how and why kids sleep. And why they don't.

I was talking with her about naps. Nap time is often one of the best times of day for any parent. This is not because you don't love your child, but rather because you still love parts of yourself too. There is something utterly delicious about the quiet and stillness in a home when you know your baby is resting peacefully. And you're off the hook for a spell.

I'm sure you wonder where you are and where you've gone off to in all of the personal clutter of raising your child. Nap time can be a moment to regain that sense of self. It's one of those hours (or 2, if you're lucky) that you get to be productive in life, but quietly and without interruption. Even if just to pay the phone bill. More, when it's for something self-preserving like writing, calling a friend, reading, or resting your body. Or for you overachievers out there, exercising.

There are days when I am utterly desperate for nap time. As my boys age and naps go out the window, my patients have helped me realize that I can still maintain it with an hour of quiet time midday on the weekend.

When it comes to running our kids into the ground at the park for the perfect nap, rationale and science are here to help us understand why it may not work. It starts with understanding what doctors call *sleep architecture*. It's the visual representation of the states of sleep: the rising and falling of our activity level, eye movements, and brain waves while we move between the stages of sleep during the night, in and out of REM sleep. Think of it as a beautiful skyline. Sleep specialists study this architecture to evaluate if we are sleeping properly and getting good-quality sleep in overnight sleep studies. The goal each and every night is to get the right amount and the right kind of sleep that refreshes, restores, and leaves us ready for the next day.

 WendySueSwanson MD @SeattleMamaDoc
Pediatric sleep expert recently explained to me that a 6 month-old's brain activity at night is the same as an 18 yo. #sleepthroughthenight

Delta-wave sleep is one part of the architecture during the night, the kind of sleep that is nearly corpse-like. It's that really deep sleep where you don't move a muscle. Real-deal rest. Think of when your child falls asleep in the car and you can carry her up and into her bed without even awaking her. Delta-wave sleep is that out-to-the-world sleep.

Not surprisingly, this delta-wave or slow-wave sleep varies depending on age. Toddlers have more delta-wave sleep than school-aged kids, adolescents, and adults. In most children (and adults), this type of deep sleep happens mostly early on in the night. However, studies have found that after athletes complete a marathon, for example, they have more delta-wave sleep and even a rebound or extra delta-wave sleep. Theoretically because they are so stinking tired.

Toddlers, if they are well-rested kids in general, will have an increase in delta-wave sleep after a long day of hard work or near marathoning. But only,

Dr Chen says, "If they are not chronically sleep deprived, are already very tired, and have a normal sleep architecture to start with.

"Many parents make the mistake of trying to run their kids into the ground to improve sleep," she notes, "and it may do just the opposite." Acute activity, like a long hike on a sunny day, really may help increase delta-wave sleep. But Dr Chen reminds, "Only in kids who are well rested prior to the activity. In kids who are chronically sleep deprived or already very tired, increasing physical activity will only rev these kids up more! And it will only reinforce their inability to fall asleep."

I translate that as running your kid into the ground may make your kid more CRAZY. You know, that tired–crazy–lunatic-like activity your toddler or preschooler (or spouse?) can have when exhausted?

So, if you're having a bad stretch of sleep and you have a wild child on your hands, don't drive off to the playground for 4½ hours of a run-into-the-ground decathlon. Let your child chill out at home, ready her for nap with a book, and keep your nap time and bedtime schedules consistent. Avoiding that park decathlon may buy you and your child a very nice nap.

44

Surviving Tantrums: The Anger Trap

Tantrums are a normal part of development. They happen most between ages 1 and 3 years, but as so many of us know, some kids are huge tantrum throwers, and some are not. Many children have more tantrums prior to and around the time of language development. Before kids are fully verbal, they're frustrated, and in that sense of frustration or hunger or dissatisfaction, tantrums can be an easy way for kids to try to get what they need.

We know tantrums are a mix of frustration and anger, but we also are learning that they are about sadness and grief too. We used to really think that tantrums started with anger and ended in sadness, but some new research says it happens all at once and that tantrums are really found to have a pattern or rhythm. The more we understand about those patterns, the more control we may feel, and the more we can help decipher when one tantrum is a real problem or is really just typical. If you've ever got any questions about your child's tantrums that you think are medically concerning, talk directly with your child's physician.

There are a couple of things that you can do with tantrums. Now, we're all told to calm down, which is probably the hardest thing to do, but you must in some ways as your anger, your frustration will only feed back to your child. Some researchers talk about this as *the anger trap*. The idea that if your kid gets angry, if you ask him questions, or if you get angry too, the anger only escalates and the tantrum prolongs. Do your best to absolutely ignore anger whenever you can.

When you ask your child questions, ask him concrete ones. Don't ask open-ended questions. Say, "Would you like the juice or the milk?" If he doesn't respond or remains angry, stop asking questions and give him a little bit of time to wind down on his own. All of us learn how to respond to our children on our own, but there is sadness and grief involved in tantrums. I know that personally, when I really started to sit down and remind myself about that, I started new techniques to help soothe my son. It really helped me, and it's really helped him.

WendySueSwanson MD @SeattleMamaDoc

Epic 2 yr old tantrum happening at our house right now. Just in case all you NYers were wondering where the screaming was coming from.

Sometimes it's really hard for us to stop tantrums. There are a couple of times when you can't ignore your child in a tantrum.

- If your child is physically at risk of running into the street or in danger, grab him tightly and hold him or make it very clear to him.
- If your child is hitting or biting, stop it immediately and make sure that you let him know that it's absolutely not acceptable by moving his body out of a situation or taking away a privilege.

Know this: tantrums do tend to get better after the age of 3. Although they don't go away entirely. Your child will do tantrums to get things that she needs normally and naturally between the ages of 1 and 3 years. Talk with your pediatrician if you're concerned about some of those behaviors. Do your best to remain calm. Use your friends and family around you to help understand how to stand back and wait for tantrums to dissolve on their own so you can come back to your child with great comfort.

We survived one of the biggest tantrums of all time in June 2012. At the Oakland, CA, airport check-in, of all places. Did you happen to hear about it? I literally had to physically hold and restrain my son from running off into moving traffic. The tantrum was cause for lots of staring and avoidance. Those stares do feel like judgment sometimes, which only makes us feel worse. In a low moment, I explained to my then-3-year-old that he was acting like an animal. I got progressively more and more embarrassed and progressively more and more frustrated. It was one of those moments we never expect and have a hard time forgetting. The forgiving, that comes easy. Have you read the book *How Do Dinosaurs Say I Love You?* That helps too. That book is delicious and captures this sentiment perfectly.

Thing is, Oden is a more of a tantrum thrower than his brother. We really didn't learn this the first time around. So when another terrible tantrum ensued soon after the airport one, I missed a meeting when I got stuck in a tornado-like tantrum and spent a big part of the weekend trying to optimize days to support my son to avoid tantrums. When it comes to tantrums, we all know we're supposed to calm down, but it's difficult. Our children find all of our hidden buttons, and they can escalate rapidly. You can't avoid every tantrum, but here are some ideas to help you survive them more gracefully.

Eight Tips to Surviving a Tantrum

- Give your child enough attention and "catch her being good." Provide specific praise in successful moments. However, don't feel that if one child tantrums more than another that you aren't providing enough attention. Personality is infused in behaviors, including tantrums.
- During a tantrum, give your child control over little things (offer small, directed choices with options rather than yes/no questions).
- Distraction. Move to a new room. Offer a safer toy. However silly, sing a song.
- Choose your battles and accommodate when you can. Sometimes you have to give in a little to settle yourself; that's OK. However, your consistency from day to day is key in reducing the level and frequency of tantrums. So is time. Although most tantrums happen in 1- to 3-year-old children, many children continue to throw tantrums into the school years.
- Know your child's limits. Obviously, some days are harder than others. Sometimes we don't get to finish the to-do list. Yesterday, someone tweeted me that Mars was in retrograde. Now I know why it was so miserable.…
- Do not ignore behaviors like hitting, kicking, biting, or throwing. Have a zero-tolerance policy.
- Set your child up for success. If tantrums peak when your child is hungry, have a healthy snack with you when you're out of the house. If they peak when your child is fatigued, prioritize sleep/nap time even if you miss things. Sometimes it's far better on all of us.
- Give yourself a break when you need it. Take turns with another parent or friend when your frustration escalates.

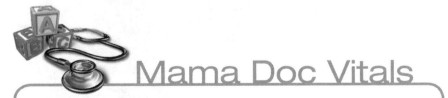

Mama Doc Vitals

Link: Anatomy of a Tantrum: http://bit.ly/mdm-tantrums

Tip: It's OK to have your own tantrum about your child's tantrums. Just wait until they're in bed! ☺

Surviving Separation Anxiety

Here's the thing about separation anxiety: it comes out of a great developmental milestone, that of *object permanence*. The ability for a child to remember that when he drops something, it's still there. So when you leave them after they've developed object permanence, some kids get really anxious. Somewhere around 9 or 10 months is when most children typically develop some separation anxiety, but we can see it develop anywhere from then until 18 months, and sometimes it can last 3 days, sometimes it lasts 3 months, and sometimes it persists even longer.

Things to Know

Separation anxiety comes at times of transition, so do your best to be really consistent. Know that after you leave, kids usually calm down and go about their daily routine. Provide your child with a transitional toy, something she can grab onto each and every time. Then provide reminders and explanations for when you'll be back. Instead of saying, "I'll be back at 3:00," tell your child you'll be back right after nap time so that she really understands when that will be, and then do your best to keep to your promises. When you say you're going to show up after nap time, do so, so that your child can really gain a sense of trust and learn how to be independent and away from you.

Separation anxiety varies WIDELY between children. Some babies become hysterical when mom is out of sight for a very short time, while other children seem to demonstrate ongoing anxiety at separations during infancy, toddlerhood, and preschool. I've got one of each in my home. The trick for surviving separation anxiety demands preparation, brisk transitions, and the evolution of time. I would suggest we parents suffer as much as our children do when we leave. Even though we are often reminded that our children stop crying within minutes of our leave-taking, how many of you have felt like you're "doing it all wrong" when your child clings to your legs, sobs for you to stay, and mourns the parting? As a working mom, separation anxiety creates questions for me. Although it is an entirely normal behavior and a beautiful sign of a meaningful attachment, separation anxiety can be exquisitely unsettling for us all. Here are facts about separation anxiety and 6 tips to improve the transitions I've learned the hard way (I've made about every mistake).

Facts About Separation Anxiety

- **Infants:** Separation anxiety develops after a child gains an understanding of object permanence. Once your infant realizes you're really gone (when you are), it may leave him unsettled. Although some babies display object permanence and separation anxiety as early as 4 to 5 months of age, most develop more robust separation anxiety at around 9 months. The leave-taking can be worse if your infant is hungry, tired, or not feeling well. Keep transitions short and routine if it's a tough day.
- **Toddlers:** Many toddlers skip separation anxiety in infancy and start demonstrating challenges at 15 or 18 months of age. Separations are more difficult when children are hungry, tired, or sick—which is most of toddler-hood! As children develop independence during toddlerhood, they may become even more aware of separations. Their behaviors at separations will be loud, tearful, and difficult to stop.
- **Preschoolers:** By the time children are 3 years of age, most clearly under-stand the effect their anxiety or pleas at separation have on us. It doesn't mean they aren't stressed, but they certainly are vying for a change. Be consistent; don't return to the room based on a child's plea, and certainly don't cancel plans based on separation anxiety. Your ongoing consistency, explanations, and diligence to return when you say you will are tantamount.

How to Survive Separation Anxiety

- **Create quick good-bye rituals.** Even if you have to do major-league-baseball–style hand movements, give triple kisses at the cubby, or provide a special blanket or toy as you leave, keep the good-bye short and sweet. If you linger, the transition time does too. So will the anxiety.
- **Be consistent.** Try to do the same drop-off with the same ritual at the same time each day you separate to avoid unexpected factors whenever you can. A routine can diminish the heartache and will allow your child to simulta-neously build trust in her independence and in you.
- **Attention:** When separating, give your child full attention, be loving, and provide affection. Then say good-bye quickly despite her antics or cries for you to stay.

- **Keep your promise.** You'll build trust and independence as your child becomes confident in her ability to be without you when you stick to your promise of return. The biggest mistake I ever made in this regard was returning to class to "visit" my son about an hour after a terrible transition. I was missing him, and although the return was well intended, I not only extended the separation anxiety, we started all over again in the process. When I left the second time (and subsequent days) it was near nuclear.
- **Be specific, child style.** When you discuss your return, provide specifics that your child understands. If you know you'll be back by 3:00 pm, tell it to your child on his terms; for example, say, "I'll be back after nap time and before afternoon snack." Define time he can understand. Talk about your return from a business trip in terms of "sleeps." Instead of saying, "I'll be home in 3 days," say, "I'll be home after 3 sleeps."
- **Practice being apart.** Ship the children off to grandma's home, schedule playdates, allow friends and family to provide child care for you (even for an hour) on the weekend. Before starting child care or preschool, practice going to school and your good-bye ritual before you even have to part ways. Give your child a chance to prepare, experience, and thrive in your absence!

It's rare that separation anxiety persists on a daily basis after the preschool years. If you're concerned that your child isn't adapting to being without you, chat with the pediatrician. Your pediatrician has certainly helped support families in the same situation and can help calm your unease and determine a plan to support both of you!

46

I Hope He Never Reads It

When Finn started preschool at age 3, they asked for items to add to their disaster kit. They wanted a gallon of water, an extra blanket, and a note to soothe Finn in case of a disaster. The thought of writing the note was simply too much for me. I hadn't given them the letter (as I was supposed to) until they asked in a follow-up email. I avoided writing it. Too tragic to thing about being separated from him in case of a major disaster and overwhelming to think of writing down something to say during the moment.

Dear Finny,

When you were just learning to talk, you used to say "kokay" instead of "OK." I really liked it. That extra "k" at the beginning of the word was all yours. You came up with it and continued it until you were almost 2½ years old. It was funny and adorable; you were the only little boy in the world I know who said it like that. In a whole school of children, I could have heard your "kokay" from across the room. Any room.

Today you say "OK" when you know you are. Say it now, Finn. You're OK.

Today is a funny day, but we are with you. Next to you, holding your hand, whispering into your right ear and squeezing your fingertips. We're nose to nose. You may not see me right now, but I'm with you. Just like the *Llama Llama* book says, even when I feel far from you, Mama is always near.

Mommy and Daddy will be with you soon. We'll smile, hug you, and squeeze you tight. We'll continue on this marvelous journey with you until we're at the edge of the sun. We'll travel to the blue sky, watch red sunsets, and dance under a bright yellow sun. We'll climb to the white tops of the mountains. You and Oden and Daddy and Mommy will have so many more journeys. You're going to have to hold on tight!

Be a brave boy until we see you. Help your friends. Listen to your teachers. Give big hugs. Be kind and sweet.

I know you'll be "kokay."

We love you more than the moon, the sun, and all the water in the ocean. See you soon, Lovey.

Love, love, love,
Mommy & Daddy

I did manage to write the letter. And then wrote one for Oden when he started too. Although writing it felt a little like I was trying to lift off part of the sky, I did have a sense of relief after it was done. Even now, I feel better knowing it's out there for him if the worse happens. I've never written something I didn't want someone to read, but I really hope he never reads this.

The Saturday Box

We're all looking for little tidbits and rituals to insert into our busy lives that actually help in that quest to have life run smoothly. I suspect the Saturday Box is one ritual worth considering.

Here's what happened in my house when I was little. When I got to school age, around third or fourth grade, my parents instituted the Saturday Box. My mom doesn't recall where she learned the idea from, but my parents put it into action at the time. Anything that was lying around for more than a reasonable amount of time in a common space in the house that wasn't supposed to be there would be deported to the Saturday Box. Anything that landed in the Saturday Box on Sunday, Monday, Tuesday, Wednesday, Thursday, or Friday, I wouldn't get back until Saturday.

The idea can help you create a great sense of responsibility for your community, your micro-community, your home with your children, from the very beginning. Can they lose rights and privileges from their own irresponsibility, and can they regain and shape how they live in an environment that's respectful to everyone around them? Can you institute a Saturday Box? Can you start by putting in toys that you find lying around the house? When you find a ball that's really supposed to have been put away earlier, can it go in the Saturday Box? Can a favorite toy go there? Can even the parent's belongings that shouldn't be left out long be put in the Saturday Box?

Use the Saturday Box to organize your house and share a sense of responsibility for your community in your home with your kids.

I'm not saying that my parents did it all right (ahem…no), but circa 1983, I think the Saturday Box exceeded expectations. Our box inspired a sense of greater responsibility and established a democratic process for cleanup in our home. Less fighting, less letdown, less guilt, and less tension. More responsibility, more ownership, and more order. The genius: the box wasn't just for my brother and me. Plenty of parental garb ended up in our Saturday Box, and the concept alone invoked a sense of equality. Not unexpectedly, we were occasionally feisty; I have a very clear memory of a family meeting being called after my father's wallet landed in the Saturday Box.…

Play

A couple of years into practicing pediatrics, I started asking a standard question, exactly the same way, to children during their 3- to 10-year-old checkups. This wasn't premeditated. Like all physicians, I go through phases of what I ask kids to elicit their experiences and beliefs, listen to their language, and observe their development. I learn a lot about my patients from what they choose to answer, in their receptive language skills (how they understand me) and their expressive skills (how they speak—fluidly, articulately, with sentences) to their cognition (how they understand concepts and theories). No child really talks as much when in the examination room as he does at home. Pediatricians know this (of course!), but these questions are a great way to learn a lot about a child's wellness and get to know my patients. It's also the part of the day I enjoy the most.

But when I started asking a standard question some years back, something became utterly clear—many children answered the exact same way. Verbatim. It continues today some 7+ years into practice.

I'd say, "What do you like to do at home?"

I expected the usual suspects. Things like, "Watch TV," "Play the DS," or "Play with princesses or dollhouses." Not that I expected stereotypes; I just expected specifics and screens because most children love them. But instead, there has been a uniform, single-word response that I get over the years. It's breathtaking. These children are all saying the exact same thing.

"Play."

One word.

It's not, "Play with_____." It's just, "Play." It has started to feel like they're defining their liberty, their freedom, or the whims of childhood. Like so many of us, they delight in the space to create, invent, imagine, and associate with others. Time to simply play.

Of course, it shouldn't be an entire surprise. The founder of Montessori herself felt that children's work was their play and that children develop through their experiences with their environment.

Delicious, isn't it?

Preschoolers and Play

Three-quarters of all preschoolers between the ages of 3 and 5 years are in child care, and more than half of them are in preschool, child care, or nursery school centers. Most children spend the majority of their waking hours after age 3 outside of their home. Many children spend very long days at school, leaving around 6:00 pm to head home. After 6:00 pm, there is little time for outdoor play.

With exercise (play) being a key strategy to prevent weight gain/obesity coupled with the reality of where children spend their day, hammering out how much children move while at school is essential. In a 2012 *Pediatrics* study, researchers interviewed child care teachers and providers from diverse centers (in Ohio) and found 3 main concerns impeding and restricting children's physical activity when in child care.

- **Injury concerns:** Children's safety was reported by parents and teachers as a main concern. Teachers, not surprisingly, felt pressure from parents not to allow children to get injured while at the centers and to restrict "vigorous" activity to avoid harm. State guidelines for safety equipment was strict, they said, but might actually be limiting children's physical activity. Many teachers felt the climbers and play equipment were boring and uninteresting and because of that, children were inventive and tried to keep it challenging by using it in unintended ways (like going up slides). As every single parent knows, the play equipment our kids like best are the ones that aren't designed for them. Rigid guidelines may be less helpful than we hope.

- **Financial concerns:** Many teachers reported that budgets restricted them from providing optimal physical activity. The equipment was noted to be very expensive ("$10,000 per climber") in some cases and not the priority of the school due to parental pressure to focus on "academics." Curriculum took precedence over gross motor play, the teachers reported. And the spaces they were afforded for play were not always optimal.

- **Focus on "academics":** This is really a story in itself, but the study found that parental pressure to prioritize academic classroom learning (pre-reading skills and colors or numbers) over active playtime was a huge concern. Teachers reported that this came from upper- and lower-income families and increased when incorporating pressures from state early-learning standards. This focus on "learning" diminished a focus on physical activity.

Instead of pointing fingers to helicopter parenting or those gunner parents who want their kids to "get ahead," I wonder if we can all be more involved in designing thoughtful days in which our children attend child care. Instead of balking at a third recess, maybe we can learn to accept that it is an essential part of our children's lives and days. New data support the notion that physical activity really does benefit learning. And in the preschool setting, we know it is an important part of health promotion. It's simple, really: we all know our quality of life improves the more time we spend outside and in play, and we certainly want our preschoolers to have the luxury to move.

Play-Based Curriculum

Play-based curriculums may be something entirely different than the play these children distill down as their uniformly favorite thing to do at home. But I believe they may complement each other. The importance of play-based learning was driven home for me after reading an opinion piece from Erika and Nicholas Christakis in 2010. Erika Christakis, an early learning teacher, and Nicholas Christakis, a professor of medicine and sociology, tackled the essence of how to prepare kids to thrive in college in a CNN article. At the time, the 2 served as housemasters to one of the residential houses at Harvard. They stated, "The real 'readiness' skills that make for an academically successful kindergartener or college student have as much to do with emotional intelligence as they do with academic preparation."

> *It's simple, really: we all know our quality of life improves the more time we spend outside and in play, and we certainly want our preschoolers to have the luxury to move.*

Children are on to something with this focus on and enjoyment of simple play. We've got to find more time, at all points in our life, to play.

Play and Recess

Children wear their self-regulation on their sleeve. Our children have good days and bad days, good spells and tough ones. One of the most important predictors of school success is the ability to control impulses. Part of how children learn to regulate their emotions and behavior is through play.

Play isn't and hasn't always held great value in the school environment. A 2009 *Pediatrics* study found that 30% of children studied had little or no significant time for recess. The study also noted that children exposed to less break time were much more likely to be black, to be from families with lower incomes and lower levels of education, to live in large cities, to be from the Northeast or South, and to attend public school, compared with those with recess.

As research is evolving about the role of play and play-based curricula, we are seeing more time for breaks during the school day. The 2009 study found that teachers rated improved behavior for children who had more break and recess time compared with those who didn't. Several studies conducted since that time find that recess (inside or outside) helped children remain attentive during classroom learning. I was shocked when my son started kindergarten in 2012 and had 3 recess periods throughout the day. He loves it, of course, and we're learning that the research backs up the design of his day!

In early 2013, a recess-promoting policy, "The Crucial Role of Recess in School," was published by the American Academy of Pediatrics (AAP). In it, the AAP defined the social-emotional, physical, nutritional, and cognitive benefits of recess. It said, "Through play at recess, children learn valuable communication skills, including negotiation, cooperation, sharing, and problem solving as well as coping skills, such as perseverance and self-control."

Erika and Nicholas Christakis' work, and the ongoing work on the benefits of play and recess for school success and emotional well-being, are gentle reminders that play-based curricula are important. Through play-based curriculum, children are reminded and required to learn to adapt and respond to other children. With play, children learn to take turns, delay gratification, negotiate conflicts, solve problems, share goals, acquire flexibility, and live with disappointment, the Christakises say.

All sounds good to me! Three cheers to those 3-recess school days out there. If only we'd had these too.

Mama Doc Vitals

Parent Power and Link: If you feel your child's preschool/school doesn't have enough outdoor or recess playtime, consider bringing this to an administrator's attention. Share with the administrator the 2013 AAP policy statement, "The Crucial Role of Recess in School" (http://bit.ly/mdm-recess).

Fact: Maria Montessori said, "Play is the work of the child," but play is so important it is also a protected child human right by the United Nations.

Tip: Unstructured, spontaneous play is one of the most important gifts we share with our children.

49

Soccer Mom

I had an unusually good time watching my boys play soccer one weekend. It has not always been easy to get our youngest on the field, and I'm not the mom who has really loved being there. There have been years of standing on the cold sideline where I didn't think the boys were getting much out of it. And there have been countless minutes on that sideline where I've been consumed, weighing the costs and benefits of the soccer class while my coffee went cold. Fortunately, something had changed recently. I'm certain it's not only me who's noticed—the boys seem differently positioned as well. Although I look in from the net and see something that seems entirely clear (a soccer field, a group of children excited and eager [or exhausted and angry], and a coach), these little boys have reminded me yet again of the diversity of vantage points we share. They really do see those green fields as a part of their future. A great coach can really make our children immensely proud and excited to be alive.

Wonder is priceless, and the pristine innocence harbored within our children often delivers moments unique to childhood. Children often hold the gift of believing that anything is possible. So often when they share this perspective we get to see a glimpse of unconfined opportunity. We're reminded of our own potential too.

Two things recently passed through my ears that I have to share. They've enhanced my soccer mom experience immensely.

One: Finn, our 6-year-old, was finishing up practice recently. As he was walking to the car, my husband said to him, "If you keep that playing up, the head coach of the Sounders is likely going to call us up and ask you to come and play for them." Apparently there was a long pause, a big beat of time. And then this: with big eyes and hope in his throat, he slowed down and looked up, his grasp just a bit firmer, and he said, "Really, Daddy?"

He really believes.

Two: After a few years of tantrums on the soccer field, our 4-year-old is finally enjoying his class. This, because of some good friends on the field and a young coach who brings delight into his eyes. After a successful practice of drills and warm-ups this weekend, his team got to play 10 minutes of scrimmage. During the scrimmage, Oden had a moment where he broke away from the pack, dribbled the ball down the length of the field, and scored a goal. He was excited, proud, but also steady. Although we've worked hard in soccer (and life) not to equate happiness with goal-scoring, he really seemed to take in the accomplishment. It was a milestone for him, and it was meaty. As we left the soccer practice, he grabbed onto his dad's hand and asked, "Dad, when I ran down the field and scored that goal, was it your BPOD [Best Part of Day]?"

This is why we keep going back. This is how the soccer mom is born again and again…

50

Inspiring Generosity in Our Children

Our 5-year-old kept forgetting to draw arms on his people at school. The lack of arms had evolved since school started in September and even came up in his fall parent-teacher conference. I found it odd—he always seems to remember that humans have arms when he draws at home. We didn't mention it to him. And when his brother got an easel for his birthday recently, Finn painted this picture. Something jumped out at me. I loved it. Not just that he remembered to put arms on this figure but the perspective it imparts. Something about this little person looks so generous and so ready to give.

It's important to help our children understand the need to give back, provide, share, and act generously. When I've thought of it before, I'd attributed our role (as parents) as role models; that is, I thought that if we act generously in front of children, they will learn how to give more freely.

A beautiful 2012 study in Public Library of Science (PLOS) ONE conducted at Yale University illuminated the complexity and maturity of our young children when it comes to giving. It made me realize that we may have to be more

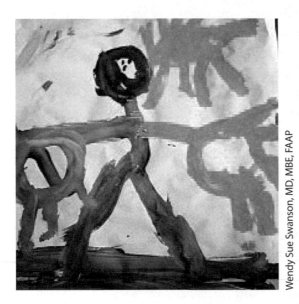

Wendy Sue Swanson, MD, MBE, FAAP

deliberate and outspoken about how and why we give. Social conditions matter when it comes to generosity and this isn't just true of adults. "Human adults are unique in that they perform what appears to be an inordinate amount of generous behavior," the study begins. Voluntary sharing really does begin as early as 2 years of age, even when "resources are easily monopolizable."

Why do children give so early and demonstrate these pro-social acts?

Researchers sought to understand how the image a child presents to others influences how much and why they give generously. Basically, they wanted to know if young children were motivated by what others thought about them when it came to their generosity. The stated that although "evidence strongly suggests that children's behavior is generally influenced by a desire to make a good impression in the eyes of others…no research to date has systematically addressed the role that audience and transparency cues play in mediating children's prosocial tendencies."

Children Are More Generous When Others Are Aware of Their Actions

Researchers set up an experiment in which 5-year-olds were tested with their peers under differing circumstances of transparency and differing audiences (ie, if others could see into the container). They set up a sticker machine that in some settings was transparent (the child giving and child receiving could see how many stickers were up for grabs), and other settings in which only the giver of stickers knew how many stickers he could give. They had children give out stickers in both settings (transparent and opaque), being able to see the recipient or not.

The results were striking: children were consistently generous only when the recipient and audience of the stickers were fully aware of the donation options (4 stickers over 1 sticker, for example). Children were notably ungenerous when the recipient of stickers couldn't see the options whatsoever. Having an audience present (seeing the recipient) and having the number of stickers be transparent affected children's decisions to give. The researchers wrote, "One striking aspect of our results is that children were considerably ungenerous in our task. Indeed, children only showed consistently prosocial behavior in our study in the condition when they could see the recipient and their allocations were fully visible; in all other conditions, children were statistically ungenerous, giving the recipient the smaller amount of stickers."

Researchers made the conclusions that children are differentially generous depending on what the recipient knows about how much you are able to give and if people are present to observe giving. Basically, children will be generous when those who are in need know how much they have to give. It seems when children can obscure their "wealth," they don't give as much away. When their friends are able to see their choices, children will give peers far more.

The take-home point for me from the study is that at a very early age, children are learning how to position themselves socially. Well before they have a handle on the sociology of their networks and what social reputation really means (normally around age 8), they think strategically about giving as a function of how they can gain a reputation with a peer as a generous citizen or pro-social agent when the recipient observes them.

How to Foster Generosity at an Early Age

Recognize that children are influenced by how their generosity is observed and understood.

Children may often think about giving under the lenses of competition. In the discussion of this paper, researchers wondered if children unintentionally thought the experiment was a competition (ie, whoever ended with the most stickers won). It is known that when competitive constructs are present, children are less generous. So are adults. Therefore, we can help young children understand when competition is present and when it isn't. If a soccer game really isn't a tally of total goals, tell children implicitly. Allow them to learn how to pass the ball and share as teammates early and often. When they are set to compete, let that be clear. But allow situations of play and giving not to be about winning too.

Children modify their behavior in response to having an audience. I suggest we help our children give to others in full view (donations to a school can drive or soup kitchen; delivering meals to families who need support) and in private or anonymously too (dropping off treats or surprises for those in your life without signing your name).

Remind children that thank-you notes are lovely but unnecessary to receive. As an adult, I've often heard people complain about not receiving a thank-you note. It's as if the reason to give a gift was to be acknowledged rather than provide something wonderful for another person. When we give gifts or lend help to others, try to help children remember why—to provide something for another. It really doesn't have to be recognized. When a thank-you card doesn't come, it doesn't make a gift any less valuable or meaningful for those who were lucky enough to receive.

51

Miserable Preschool Drop-offs

Sometimes it feels like we've got it all in control—a new school, a new schedule, a return back to work obligations. We can set the alarm early, burn the midnight oil, pack the school lunch ahead of time, rise up and meet the challenge. Sometimes it all works and everyone thrives.

Sometimes, no.

Sometimes it is simply miserable to leave our children behind and trudge off to work.

Miserable.

It doesn't mean we don't care about our jobs or that we lack compassion or a passion, intent, or drive to serve. It really can mean that we just love our children.

A drop-off circa 2012 at preschool sticks with me. I'd woken up early to prepare lunch, get Finn up for car pool pickup, and ready myself for work. But something about the start didn't feel right. A little twinge in my heart had me muttering, "Sometimes you just wake up feeling sad." I was missing the boys before they were gone.

I really didn't want to be a working mom that day.

I puttered around the kitchen, soaked up the boys at breakfast, and did my best to prop my chin up. It was my turn to drop off Oden, our 3-year-old, at school. He skipped in the front door, headed straight to the cubby to pop off his shoes, and I signed him in. Just then, the bomb dropped.

As if he could sense my hesitation about the day, he literally death-gripped my legs and looked up. "Pleeeeeeeeaase don't leave me here, Mommy."

That was all it took. He sobbed; I sobbed. Miserable mess—we've been doing this for years—why the salt in my wound today? At minute mark 3 or 4, I realized I was doing no one any good sticking around. I offered up a Kissing Hand, asked for one in return (and was rejected by him), and headed off to the car. The day unfolded as one of those days where the ceiling just seems a bit lower.

Sometimes, it's miserable to separate from our children. Separation anxiety may be my diagnosis too at times. But thank goodness it fills the reuniting with magic.

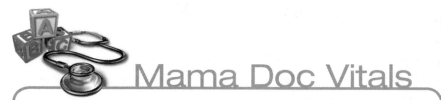

Mama Doc Vitals

Book: *The Kissing Hand* is a delicious little story that offers up a practice for you and your child at drop-off. Pick up a copy or visit the library to learn more.

Truth: Miserable drop-offs can happen at any age. Sometimes they are just a sign of a wonderful bond.

WendySueSwanson MD @SeattleMamaDoc

Had the most miserable, sad preschool drop-off of life. Leaving for #SXSW with a v heavy heart. #worklifebalance

52

No More "Clean Plate Club"

Some new advice allows us to do less, not more. Turns out, 2013 research finds that controlling parenting styles may hinder children's healthy eating habits. New data published find that not only are controlling, food-related parenting practices common, they aren't helping teens maintain a healthy weight. In the *Pediatrics* study, researchers found that parents often encourage teens of healthy weight to finish all of their food, providing pressure to eat, while parents of overweight teens ban some foods and encourage restriction. Neither practice is proven to improve teens' habits or their health.

We really want our children to self-regulate their energy intake (food), and mounting evidence reports that controlling habits hinder this essential skill.

Four Golden Eating Rules

1. **Divide responsibilities.** Parents have the job of purchasing and serving healthy food. Infants, children, and teens have to choose what and how much to eat of the food that's offered. We can enhance nutritionist Ellyn Satter's division of responsibilities that directs us each to have our own roles. Every parent knows that you can't force a child to eat; the best thing to do is stop trying. Let mealtime be about feeding your body. If your children don't eat much, wait until the next meal to offer food. Children eat for themselves, not for their parents. Turn the TV off and let children feel their fullness when it arrives.

2. **Eat when your body is hungry. Stop when your body is full.** Infants do this naturally when breastfeeding and starting solids. We have to do our best to maintain that natural habit throughout toddlerhood to the teen years. This skill of responding to natural hunger and normal cues of satiety can be a huge asset for children for their entire lives. Do your best to stop engineering how much your children eat and let them learn to feel necessities.

> *We really want our children to self-regulate their energy intake (food), and mounting evidence reports that controlling habits hinder this essential skill.*

3. **Don't make children "clean the plate."** There's absolutely no reason to provide pressure for children with normal development and health to eat. Don't reward children for finishing their dinner with more food (ie, dessert), as children will often eat past their fullness. New research also finds that using smaller plates can help control portion sizes and ultimately will reduce the number of calories eaten. The benefit: it will also trigger less need to ask them to clean their plate; they'll do so naturally on a smaller plate.

4. **Eat together.** The most potent education we give our children comes from our modeling habits and behaviors we think are most important. Eat together with children at meals from infancy until they leave home. Make a goal for at least one meal a day, and it doesn't need to be dinner. There's no reason to cook special food for your children. Involve them in any part of meal preparation you can, eat the same foods, and share your love of eating.

53

Digital Sabbatical and Digital Sabbath

I can't say enough about the power of being unplugged. Digital Sabbaths have become important.

It's only this past 5 years that we all find ourselves entirely consumed and surrounded by our screens. Somehow we have to carve out breaks. I'm terrible about putting my phone down, so I've had to be more ritualized about taking breaks.

I love the luxury of living in 2013. I get to read bedtime stories via Skype or Google+ Hangouts when I'm 2,000 miles away on a business trip. I capture my boys at school, in the yard, or at the soccer game with my iPhone. I'm not someone who's going to point a finger about your device (unless you're driving).

But breaks? They have been saviors for me.

I've done a number of digital Sabbaths these past few years. Not enough, of course, but a few. The concept: take 24 hours off-line from Friday at sundown through Saturday at sunset. You don't use a phone, text, or log onto a computer. You don't enter an online network. When I've done them I don't blog, tweet, or use Facebook or LinkedIn with anyone. I don't answer or read e-mails. As a digital doctor, that's a toughie, but I've done it.

And the breaks are divine and restorative.

The lesson is simple, of course. Twenty-four hours without digital distractions are exceptionally bright. The loss from being disconnected online is overwhelmingly surpassed by the gains acquired with being present off-line. The unplugged time is an utter luxury for me in the time of exceptional connectivity and work online.

I said this after my very first digital sabbatical in 2010: "There's nothing I would do to reverse my time offline. It was rich and it's solidified the need to establish a new goal to make time for a more frequent digital sabbatical. I want to seek solace routinely from the deluge of content, information, exceptional wisdom, and friendship I gain while online and return to the spaces without distraction that house the same things."

I noticed how different I was when detached from my beloved phone.

I was different on my arrival home. More present with the boys, making different decisions, and moving at a new pace. I was letting time unfold instead of folding pieces of life into time. No racing around, checking my pocket, drafting e-mails in my head, writing and rewriting blogs.

The New York Times writer Matt Richtel has written about the effect of our digital world on our lives, our brains, and our functionality in a series called "Your Brain on Computers." Although my iPhone, laptop, and other devices allow me to constantly contribute to and learn from the (non)medical world around me, Matt Richtel points out, "…when people keep their brains busy with digital input, they are forfeiting downtime that could allow them to better learn and remember information, or come up with new ideas."

Just think of what I'd know if I didn't spend so much time here.

Joking aside, Matt Richtel followed a group of neuroscientists on a 3-day remote excursion without digital technology as they evaluated their changed attention and processing speeds. What they describe (a clutter-free slowdown) is exactly how I felt. And I didn't read the article until I returned home! Relaxation is a powerful thing. Yet many of us have none of it, particularly while raising young children.

Mr Richtel has written about the increasingly large debate surrounding attention, distraction, and the speed at which we live and process information in the 21st century. This urgent-get-right-back-to-you-status-update lifestyle comes at great costs. Even though occasionally it reaps great rewards too.

Certainly starved for some more downtime, this unexpected, un-wired weekend was illustrative. I know I'm out of balance.

Tips for Digital Breaks

- Take a 24-hour digital sabbatical whenever you can. If you break the fast, don't beat yourself up. Even 6 hours off-line is great.
- Align yourselves. Convince your partner (or teen!) to take the 24-hour break with you. I've found that buddying up improves my success and stamina.
- When on vacation or at an important event, consider turning off your Wi-Fi and access to networks to decrease the urge to just "check in." However weak it sounds, many people who do this enjoy the decreased urge.

You may want the phone around for coordination or for taking photos, but you likely don't need the Internet.

WendySueSwanson MD @SeattleMamaDoc

I'm taking a digital sabbatical. Will be back shortly! #WorkLifeBalance employs strong intent and demands scheduled diligence.

Dr Google

For practicing physicians, there's a tricky balance in believing that the Internet can help save lives.

I'm a doctor who encourages families to look up health information online and who believes that technology will afford improved partnerships. Yet, when we're in the old-fashioned examination room, there isn't always a place for the Internet. Many clinics block video-streaming sites and don't allow for traditional e-mail exchanges between clinicians and patients. It's hard to "send" patients information discussed during the visit. In the 10 or 20 minutes we have together, time is precious. Truth be told, health care remains wary of doctors and patients communicating when they're not in the exam room. Most insurers won't pay for electronic communication between patients and their clinicians, so doctors are often forced to bring you into the office to provide expertise. New data today may help change this paradigm. Reality is, many of us are using the Internet as a tool for health care.

For at least one-third of American adults, the Internet is a diagnostic tool.

Yet, it's not just insurers who may be wary of online information. Recently I read a patient review (online) from a parent who was frustrated I'd encouraged them to read the content on my blog. The comment implied that perhaps I was "pushing it." And that's the tricky part—when I first started writing the blog, I was bashful to mention it in clinic. I wanted patients to feel comfortable, NOT pressured. But now that I have more than 400 blog posts showcasing research and pediatric health information, it's tantamount that I share it. I mean, if I'm in the midst of a 15-minute visit and we touch on topics like getting a carbon monoxide monitor, the choking game, the Tdap shot, and the effects of TV on a child's developing brain, how could I not augment a parent's or teen's understanding by offering more information online?

Numerous studies find that what parents learn in the exam room with doctors isn't retained. That's where Dr Google comes in.

> *For at least one-third of American adults, the Internet is a diagnostic tool.*

Like any other pediatrician, I want parents to know as much about their children's health as possible. The Internet is another tool. I firmly believe that the future job description for primary care doctors will include filtering and offering up great online sites for parents to read, search, and ask questions about their children's health. Thing is, many people are using Dr Google before the visit.

Dr Google and Going in to See the Real Doctor

New information in 2013 from the Pew Research Center demonstrated some realities about our relationship with Dr Google. The center surveyed more than 3,000 Americans, inquiring about their relationship with health information-seeking online in the previous year. Some of what they found follows:

One in 3 US adults (and nearly half of college-educated adults) use the Internet to diagnose themselves or someone else they care about. After these "online diagnosers" have finished a search, their clinician is more likely than not to confirm their suspicions. So it's not just that people go online to diagnose a medical problem or concern; they take what they learn online and head in to see their physician. Nearly half (46%) say that what they find online made them feel that they needed to see a clinician. Further, 41% of those who went into the doctor's office had the diagnosis they found online confirmed by their physician.

Women are more likely than men to go online looking for a diagnosis for themselves or a loved one. You're also more likely to go online to diagnose if you're a young adult, white, have a college degree, or live in a home earning more than $75,000.

There are some issues, though, outside of the obvious concerns about quality of information. One in 4 people looking online for health information report that they have hit a pay wall. This means patients are blocked from information they'd like to see. Some can go on Twitter and ask a clinician to send the study of interest, but not most. Of those who get blocked, surprisingly 83% of people who couldn't get into the medical research they wanted continued to look for the information elsewhere. Turns out all of our late-night online searching has made us resourceful online diagnosers!

Seventy-seven percent of people reported using a search engine first for finding out about a potential diagnosis. Only 13% of people went directly to a health site first (something like Seattle Children's, HealthyChildren.org,

MayoClinic.com, or WebMD). And not surprisingly, only 1% said they surveyed their social network (ie, Facebook) first.

To be honest, nothing about these data surprised me, even though the Pew Research Center mentioned that this was the first time anyone had measured these findings in a straightforward, national survey.

My clinical practice and experience is likely skewed (by age, education, socioeconomics, and race). The number of people who reported going online to diagnose (35% overall) seemed lower than I would have expected. Most parents whom I talk with in clinic have been online to read about their child's development, immunizations, sleep, or diet at some point. Many new parents do significant amounts of reading even before the baby arrives! In my opinion, we forget that when we're reading about preventive strategies (eg, safe sleep, vaccines, ways to feed a baby, ways to protect babies from chemicals, ways to avoid the flu), we're reading about health. Often people think about health care as only problem resolution—we only think we're doing medical "research" online when we're curing illness, anxiety, or pain. In my world, prevention is key. The Internet is one of those keys.

Online Search With Google

I wasn't surprised to see that 80% of online diagnosers used a search engine (eg, Google, Bing) first when looking for a diagnosis. We're impatient and busy, and search engines provide rapid responses—no wonder we all start there! Even in the examination room with patients, I often will start with a search engine when a family and I seek to find information.

I think the complexity and trick of serving patients well is in the next step, what comes next—AFTER online diagnosers peruse search engine results. Which site you click on next is telling and likely will have lasting effects on the quality of information you find. That's where we physicians need to be useful—we need to help our patients know where to go for quality, research-based, data-backed advice.

Parents Learn Much About Their Children Online

Most parents learn about their children's health outside of the pediatrician's office. I think it's more common that a parent looks things up online when worried about something new, like a lump on an infant's head or a new rash. In my experience, nearly 1 in 3 or maybe 1 in 2 of my patients will tell me that they have been online in those sick visits. Contrastingly, in visits for things like cough, ear infection, or colds, parents rarely report that they have been online.

Tips for Online Diagnosers

- Keep a bread-crumb trail as best you can. When we're online, we forget where we go and often don't know who we're listening to. Confusion comes in when families don't remember where they have been gathering information and become confused by myths, personal anecdotes, and stories that lead them astray. Everything on the Internet is clearly not in our best interest as parents. One solution: print things out or refer to specific links with your physician when you're in to see him or her so you can look online information up together.

- Look for advice from experts (psychologists, physicians, researchers). As parents and patients, we don't make all of our health decisions using science, but when we have the opportunity to use solid data to steer decisions, we want the correct sources. Your doctor can help vet the online voices to which you tune. Ask your pediatrician or clinician what sites he or she trusts the most.

- Look for sites affiliated with academic medical centers or health care institutions. Often those sites vet and scrutinize content with their expert researchers and clinicians. I tend to encourage families to avoid sites heavily laden with advertising, as I've learned that content on those sites can sometimes be edited to meet requirements in tone, scope, or opinion by advertisers.

- It's my opinion that the last thing we physicians should do is shut down our patients' online searches. It's a new world; we must join our patients online because nearly half of many groups are using Dr Google to diagnose. We must guide families to trusted and valuable voices and then help confirm or redirect the results of their online learning.

- Lastly, take a peek at my list of doctors and researchers to follow online and on Twitter in "Online Resources for Parents" starting on page 373!

Part 3

Immunizations

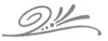

WHAT'S THE REAL STORY ON VACCINES?

When we have children, we all hear a lot about vaccines and vaccine safety. It's critical for your child's health that you know the important facts. The bottom line is that vaccines preserve life and livelihood; the science is clear on that.

DO WE REALLY NEED VACCINES?

ABSOLUTELY! It's a fact that vaccines save lives on an individual and massive scale.

Cases per Year in 20th Century	PERCENT DECREASE		2010 Reported Cases
29,005	Smallpox	100%	0
21,053	Diphtheria	100%	0
16,316	Polio (paralytic)	100%	0
152	Congenital rubella syndrome	100%	0
530,217	Measles	>99%	63
47,745	Rubella	>99%	5
20,000	*Haemophilus influenzae*	99%	246
162,344	Mumps	98%	2,612
580	Tetanus	96%	26
200,752	Pertussis	86%	27,550

And they are significantly reducing many of today's most worrisome diseases.

Since 1995, when the varicella shot was approved for routine use, chickenpox-related deaths have diminished

97%

POX PARTIES

(Yet some families still try to get chickenpox "naturally" at pox parties.)

In June 2013, the Centers for Disease Control and Prevention (CDC) reported that human papillomavirus (HPV) infection in girls aged 14–19 decreased from

7.2% 2006 > **3.6%** 2010

presumably because of the HPV vaccine.

THE BIG QUESTIONS

DO VACCINES CAUSE AUTISM?

NO!

The myth that the MMR vaccine causes autism came from a now-discredited study.

Numerous scientific studies have shown NO association between MMR immunization among young children and an increase in autism.

DO THEY CAUSE MORE HARM THAN GOOD?

NO!

EFFECTS OF CATCHING DISEASE

MEASLES

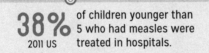

38%
2011 US

of children younger than 5 who had measles were treated in hospitals.

Can lead to pneumonia, lifelong brain damage, deafness—even death

 1-3 out of 1,000 US children who get measles will die.

MUMPS

Though usually mild, it can cause serious problems, including meningitis and deafness, and can be deadly.

RUBELLA

Most dangerous for a fetus: can cause miscarriage or birth defects like deafness, intellectual disability, and heart defects

85/100 babies born to mothers who had rubella in the first trimester will have a birth defect.

IN CONTRAST, ANY POTENTIAL SIDE EFFECTS FROM GETTING THE VACCINE ARE RARE AND USUALLY MILD, SUCH AS ALLERGIC REACTIONS OR FEVER.

95% More than 95% of people who receive MMR shots become immune to all 3 diseases—AMAZING!

ALTERNATIVE SCHEDULES

Discuss any questions about vaccination schedules with your pediatrician. Note that

Nearly **90%** of parents follow the physician-recommended schedule.

55% of families on alternative schedules ultimately get all recommended vaccines but on a delayed schedule.

 Delaying vaccines increases your child's risk for serious diseases such as measles and pertussis.

Many families do not use scientific data when determining their own vaccine schedule.

Vaccines are extensively studied; schedules shouldn't be adjusted without consideration for the science.

SOURCES
* www.cdc.gov/vaccines/vpd-vac/measles/faqs-dis-vac-risks.htm * www.aapredbook.org/content/1/SEC8/SEC9.extract *
* www.aap.org/immunization/families/faq/vaccinestudies.pdf *
* www.cdc.gov/vaccines/hcp/patient-ed/conversations/prevent-diseases/provider-resources-factsheets-infants.html *
* http://seattletimes.com/text/2021368963.html * http://pediatrics.aappublications.org/content/early/2011/09/28/peds.2011-0400.abstract?papetoc *
* www.bmj.com/content/342/bmj.c7452 *

Part 3
Immunizations

Introduction

Thoughts on Vaccines and Alternative Schedules

In this part of the book, I share some stories and information about the vaccine schedule, vaccine safety, and fear surrounding getting children immunized. It's clearly not intended to be comprehensive; rather, this section is designed to touch on issues and research that doesn't get the light I feel it deserves. I also hope it allows you to think about new ways to read about vaccines online and resources for you to use when you have questions along the way.

You'll hear most pediatricians say, "If it were my child, I'd get all the recommended shots." The advice is easy to give, as most pediatricians believe there is simply no safer way to care for children. Yet some parents are hesitant to take that advice.

Of course, a certain sense of unease is normal when it comes to our children's shots. On the days my boys get immunized, I feel queasy too when I think about the pain and anxiety that comes with getting poked with a sharp needle, sometimes more than once. But some parents worry even more about the safety and efficacy of vaccines, and often for what seem like very logical reasons. We can't be expected to understand vaccine science as elegantly as experts who have studied infectious diseases and vaccines for a lifetime, so we approximate expertise by following the experts' recommendations. Trouble is, lately it can feel like we shouldn't—there are so many voices telling us to question the rules.

In my opinion, following are the main factors that have conspired to lead parents astray and cause us to become more hesitant about vaccines:

Powerful Storytelling

We've all heard stories about the harms of vaccines. And I'm not just talking about celebrities. I'm talking about your neighbor's sister's nephew, or your cousin, or your college roommate's son, or even your own brother. We hear stories of side effects that may or may not reflect the truth. We hear stories about being "natural," as if being unimmunized is more organic. Often, patients' or parents' interpretation of side effects may not be causally linked. The side effects they see may be coincidence.

The thing about the stories we hear is that the truth can play second fiddle to emotion. When we hear vaccine stories, we feel their emotion and are reminded of our sense of vulnerability for our family's health. And this brews earnest and understandable worry. It's hard to grab onto facts when stories circulate. It's hard to forget or unlearn myths or anecdotes that warp and change when passed along.

Secondary to mounting concerns about vaccine safety over the last decade, the Institute of Medicine (IOM)—the watchdogs of medicine—reviewed more than 1,000 research papers on vaccine science and safety in 2013. This was its final conclusion.

> *"This report is the most comprehensive examination of the immunization schedule to date. The IOM committee uncovered no evidence of major safety concerns associated with adherence to the childhood immunization schedule."*

Unfortunately, the IOM report doesn't tell an evocative story about one specific child. The remarkable feat of reviewing 1,000 studies that confer the safety of vaccines gets lost.

What I want more than anything else in my life is for my children to thrive. I want them to survive everything. I want them to die of old age. I suspect you feel exactly the same way.

So when we hear news reports, stories, or even "alternative" physicians hesitating about immunizations, we worry and we remember. I certainly heard about the doctor who practices just blocks from my office who doesn't "believe" in the flu shot. You've probably heard about doctors who care for celebrities or the very wealthy and use alternative vaccine schedules. These stories make us wonder—is someone else getting better care? Is that schedule more privileged?

Problem is, we rarely hear stories about the harms associated with vaccine-preventable disease or the harms of waiting on vaccines, so our emotion may be informed in a lopsided way.

> *What I want more than anything else in my life is for my children to thrive. I want them to survive everything. I want them to die of old age. I suspect you feel exactly the same way.*

In my practice, I want to connect parents with true experiences of illness so they can recognize the rationale for getting shots. So I tell families about the infant who died from pertussis at 1 month of age just miles from my clinic. She was too young to be immunized, and her family and community weren't comprehensively immunized against whooping cough at the time of her birth. I try to detail stories of babies and children who suffered consequences of pneumococcal, influenza, polio, and *Haemophilus influenzae* type b infections that I've seen in my training and practice. I don't tell these story to scare but rather to balance the lopsided way stories circulate about vaccines and safety. We have to share these stories so we all get a fair chance at understanding.

Families may avoid going to see the physician because of the stories they hear. Watercooler conversations create hesitancy in us all to trust our child's doctor and the advice of experts who lead organizations like the Centers for Disease Control and Prevention or the American Academy of Pediatrics, who together make the vaccine schedule. The experts making the immunization schedules know far more about vaccine safety than you or me. And they have children too. I do trust them, and I, like you, will keep asking questions when I don't understand.

Parental Instinct

As mothers and fathers, one of the universal gifts we're given is our instinct. I love to use it and love to feel it when making decisions for my children. Think about the moment you knew your child was sick before anyone else or the moment you came up with a solution like diving into the wood chips to catch your son on play equipment just before he fell. It's natural that our instinct would lead us to believe that the act of intervention (inserting a needle into our child's leg) is more dangerous than the act of nonintervention (not immunizing your child).

There's no wonder we're uneasy when the doctor asks the nurse to inject our child 5 times at a well-child visit. I would suggest we're very normal when we feel unease. But the hesitations that come from this instinct have potential repercussions. We have to remember that the act of being left unvaccinated and unprotected also comes with risk. For our children *and* those we love.

Vulnerable populations of people live everywhere. Children with suppressed immune systems, children on chemotherapy, the elderly, and those unable to get vaccines. When we protect our children, we also protect our friends, family, and community.

WendySueSwanson MD @SeattleMamaDoc

No vaccines work 100% of the time. Once immunized, some are still susceptible. We're always dependent on our neighbors for protection.

The Internet

The World Wide Web gives us access to tremendous knowledge. We live in a time of spectacular medical breakthroughs and unparalleled connectivity online. I spend the majority of my time online now, helping to share health information and improve the way we can partner to care for our children. We live in this time when our children are protected from infectious diseases that historically killed handfuls of our relatives. But we also live in a time where these concrete medical successes can by drowned out by one well-told story. One beautiful, articulate, powerful mom can tell a story we'll never forget. And sometimes these stories may leave us feeling responsible to learn a lot online, all on our own.

Often I think parents feel like they are supposed to be doing their own research on vaccines. It's as if, over the last 20 years, pediatricians and infectious disease experts aren't the trusted partner we want. In my opinion, that's a missed opportunity for trust. I don't think you have to do research online, but you certainly can and, in my mind, should be encouraged to do so. When you do go online, you want to be really thoughtful about who has written what you're reading. Does the author have expertise, or is it just a story? Do you leave a breadcrumb trail when you click around on the Internet? Do you know where you were when you were learning what you did?

I certainly often have no recollection of all the places I've been online in an evening.

Paul Offit, MD, FAAP, chief of infectious diseases at the Children's Hospital of Philadelphia, reminded me, "You can't Google vaccines and know just as much" as an expert. Although many of us think we can. The Pew Research Center has found that 80% of all Americans who use the Internet are searching for health information online. When this book went to press, we knew that 35% of Americans were going online to self-diagnose—it's hard not to, and I believe it should be encouraged. But we really do need to know where to go. Most parents are online daily, learning about their children's opportunities (and health) in social networks and on blogs and Web sites. I believe there is great information to be discovered.

Reality is, there is potentially a crack in the armor in our online searching. The difference resides in the quality of research we do as parents versus the research that happens at academic medical centers. We have to be careful about what information we collect online and what conclusions we draw. Whenever possible, if you read information online that changes what you'll do for your child, tag it or print it out and bring it in with you to the next visit to see the pediatrician. Partner with the doctor and see what he or she thinks about what you've read.

In my opinion, even though I went to medical school and got pediatric training, I still don't know enough to make a vaccine schedule for my own children. Fortunately, medical school taught me in whom to trust and how to value those who help make the immunization schedule.

The experts who make the schedule for the chickenpox vaccine have had far more training than me. For example, when making the schedule for chickenpox shots, experts reviewed more than 300 research studies pertaining to varicella (the virus that causes chickenpox). The research that we can do online may not compare.

Since 1995, when the varicella shot was approved for routine use, deaths due to chickenpox have diminished 97%. However, some families still try to get chickenpox "naturally" by attending pox parties. In 2011, we learned about Facebook groups coalescing around claims to improve immunity by having lollipops licked by kids with chickenpox sent through the mail, a potentially dangerous and simultaneously unhelpful act (chickenpox would be unlikely to survive the transit). I remain incredulous that a parent would chose a stranger's lollipop over a safe and well-tested vaccine, but this also reminds me how scared many of us are about getting our kids the recommended shots. Chickenpox parties on Facebook and Web sites committed to scaring families by purporting that vaccines cause autism all feed the fire of myth and misinformation about immunizations. And that's where the Internet simply doesn't serve us as well as it can and will as time unfolds.

No Memory of Disease

One reason many families feel "safer" delaying or refusing vaccines is a hampered memory of real disease. It typically doesn't feel like infectious diseases are knocking on the front door. And in general, most of them aren't. Most of the diseases we now prevent with vaccines really are rare. But the issue of waning community immunity is real; this is proved by more frequent outbreaks of measles and deaths from diseases like pertussis and influenza.

To be clear, the reasons for pertussis outbreaks are varied. It's not just unimmunized communities; more research shows that our children's immunity wanes after their fifth dose of the shot protecting them from pertussis (DTaP). Further, we know that the shot only protects about 80% of those who get the vaccine. And lastly, we know that since we switched to a vaccine with less side effects (DTaP versus DTP) in the 1990s, the immunity created from the shot has less lasting effects. All these factors, in addition to those who are under-immunized, may set our communities up for more outbreaks of disease. It's therefore even more important that all of our community members get immunized to protect us all.

> *You don't want to wait for epidemics to motivate families to immunize.*

In my experience in practice during the 2012 whooping cough epidemic we had in Washington, the reminder of real disease became a huge motivator for families to be immunized and protect their babies and children from whooping cough. Families made special visits to immunize all members in their home, and many families restricted visitors for their newborns who didn't have Tdap vaccination. Families reminded of disease became vigilant and fierce purveyors of public health initiatives.

You don't want to wait for epidemics to motivate families to immunize.

My mother has talked to me about what my grandmother did to shield her and my 3 uncles against polio before the first vaccines were given. They were living in a time of fear, with polio circling around communities and causing paralysis in their neighbors and friends. My mom reflects that it was an incredibly easy decision, I suspect, to get the polio vaccine. Now, most of us don't know much about polio. We're closing in on worldwide eradication, thanks to efforts from groups like the Bill & Melinda Gates Foundation. So when I'm talking with parents of newborns stressing a need for the polio vaccine, the equation of risk may not compute.

Sometimes I think about my grandma, who died from cancer, when talking with families about the safety of the human papillomavirus (HPV) vaccine for adolescents. If she only knew that girls and boys entering junior high school could be immunized against a cancer-causing virus or that at birth, every baby gets a start on preventing hepatitis B, a virus that can lead to cancer of the liver, she would be mesmerized by the opportunity afforded by these advanced vaccines. And I suspect she would be equally shocked to know that some families refuse the vaccines.

Advice from Non-vaccine Experts

I'm not a vaccinologist. But I am a pediatrician and mom who asks a lot of questions and helps parents get connected to answers. Truth be told, most of my knowledge about risks, side effects, effectiveness, and science of vaccines has come from my advocacy work and writing alongside my experience working as a general pediatrician. I've had to look up lots of studies and information on vaccines to help parents understand.

> *If you talk with a physician who you don't think is informed about vaccines, take it on yourself to provide information you've discovered or concerns or questions you hold.*

However, some physicians may claim expertise when they don't have it. For instance, back in 2007, Robert Sears, MD, FAAP, published a book on vaccines. Targeting families who were concerned about vaccine safety, he came up with a delayed schedule to assuage fear. However, no scientific study has ever supported that waiting to get a vaccine has any benefit. All an alternative schedule does is simply increase the time a child is vulnerable for infection while providing the same risks when children do get immunized. Vaccine experts often go so far as to call alternative schedules, "The worst possible schedules." You get absolutely no benefit from waiting and no less risk.

Frankly, I think Dr Sears' idea just feels better to some parents even though there is no safety record for his alternative vaccine schedule (the book's readers may not know that a measles infection was transmitted by one of Dr Sears' patients during a 2008 measles outbreak in California). The further we get from the time when British citizen Andrew Wakefield erroneously claimed that MMR causes autism, and the farther we get from Jenny McCarthy being on *Oprah* claiming the same thing, the fewer of Dr Sears' books I see in my office. However, his book carries huge weight among families who remain worried. Reality is, that group of parents is becoming a smaller minority. Less than 10% of families recently interviewed about using an alternative schedule said they used one like his.

> *An alternative schedule is an untested schedule.*

If you talk with a physician who you don't think is informed about vaccines, take it on yourself to provide information you've discovered or concerns or questions you hold. I learn from patients frequently when it comes to vaccine information—on rumors or statistics they inquire about. Do the same for your doctor if you're confused or feel he or she isn't aware of something you've learned or read. Your physician will know how to look up needed answers for you when questions arise.

We live in a time of great fortune. Immunizations save many of our lives—silently. And as we work to sort through the stories, regain trust in our experts, and manage our instincts, I believe we will see fewer families using alternative schedules and hopefully more of us connected with the information we need to make great decisions for our children's health. Perhaps we'll hone the schedule even better to protect our children as we understand more as science evolves.

We all want the same thing: healthy children and healthy communities.

Cocoon a Newborn: Only an E-mail Away

In 2012, Washington declared that whooping cough (pertussis) had reached epidemic levels. It had already reached epidemic levels in California back in 2010. These pockets of rising infection and epidemic level increase risk for new babies. Infants are most susceptible to life-threatening infections from whooping cough and have very little immunity.

In clinic I've been urging new parents to *cocoon* their babies; that is, provide a family of surrounding protection by having every single child and adult immunized against whooping cough, influenza, and other vaccine-preventable illnesses. By surrounding a baby with only immunized people, you cocoon the baby against serious infections.

Whooping cough is a highly infectious respiratory illness spread by sneezing and coughing that can be deadly to young infants. Getting a tetanus, diphtheria, acellular pertussis (Tdap) shot is the best way to avoid getting whooping cough. Amid an epidemic, we worry most about newborns because they are most vulnerable to complications and lack vaccine protection. If every child and adult who surrounds a newborn gets a Tdap shot, the likelihood of the baby getting whooping cough approaches zero.

Most newborns get whooping cough from their family or adults around them. That's where an e-mail comes into play.

You may have to be fairly Mama/Papa Bear about this. You'll have to show some strength to create a very safe home, even when it feels somewhat over the top. As I said to a number of families, "It only seems entirely over-the-top nuts until we lose another newborn to pertussis." Being smart now will save lives.

Make a new rule. *No visits with a newborn until all visitors have had the Tdap shot. Even grandparents.*

WendySueSwanson MD @SeattleMamaDoc

Newborn died of pertussis in Seattle area on December 13th. All parents, sibs, grandparents, & visitors of newborn babies need a Tdap shot!

Write an E-mail to Family and Friends to Explain

Here is a sample e-mail for you to use/copy/share, written by a friend of mine.

Hi there,

We are hoping we get to see you and introduce you to our new baby sometime in the next few months!

Due to the pertussis epidemic around here and the fact that flu incidence is peaking, I am being a stickler about only having visitors who have had the flu shot and Tdap vaccine. We just got back from our doctor, who emphasized how important this is, as both—especially pertussis—are very serious for infants. A Tdap shot should be completed 2 weeks before hanging out with a newborn.

You can get both at your doctor's office and at many pharmacies that do vaccines. Thanks for understanding!

What Is Whooping Cough? And What About the Tdap Shot?

Whooping cough is a bacterial infection caused by the bacteria pertussis. You catch whooping cough by being exposed to someone with the cough who spreads bacteria into the air. The bacteria comes into the airways, causing inflammation and spasm; this irritation leads to a cough. When a baby or child is short of breath, he inhales deeply and quickly between coughs, and when he does so, he sometimes can cause a "whooping" sound—which is how whooping cough got its common name. In older children, the "whoop" sound is more common and causes them to cough in fits or to the point of vomiting. In babies and toddlers, it may not be accompanied by the "whoop."

Infants younger than 1 year (and specifically younger than 2 months) are at greatest risk of developing severe breathing problems and life-threatening illness from whooping cough. And although we want to protect everyone from whooping cough, we worry most about babies.

To protect against whooping cough, infants and children get the diphtheria, tetanus, acellular pertussis (DTaP) vaccine. They get it first at 2, 4, and 6 months of age, then at 15 to 18 months and 4 years of age. After the dose at 15 months, most toddlers are thought to be immune to whooping cough.

Children 11 years and older and all adults get the tetanus, diphtheria, acellular pertussis (Tdap) vaccine.

Tdap is a shot necessary for all adults and children starting at age 11 years that protects against infections caused by tetanus, diphtheria, and pertussis. Because of increasing reports of whooping cough and increased infant deaths in the last few years, we are working hard to protect infants, children, adolescents, and adults from pertussis. Most importantly, we want to protect our newborns from being exposed to or contracting whooping cough. Whooping cough is most dangerous and devastating (occasionally fatal) for newborns and infants younger than 6 months.

If you are around a newborn, it's essential that you've had a Tdap shot at least once as an adult.

Keep in mind that even fully vaccinated adults can get pertussis. Most data show that about 80% of us who are immunized are protected, but over time, the protection wears off. If you are sick with a cold or cough and are caring for infants, check with your health care professional about what's best for your situation.

When to Call the Pediatrician: Pertussis infection starts out acting like a cold. You should consider the possibility of whooping cough if the following conditions are present:

- The child is a very young infant who has not been fully immunized or has had exposure to someone with a chronic cough or the disease.
- The child's cough becomes more severe and frequent or her lips and fingertips become dark or blue.
- She becomes exhausted after coughing episodes, eats poorly, vomits after coughing, and/or looks sick.

How to Protect Your Family Against Whooping Cough

- The best way to prevent pertussis (whooping cough) is to get vaccinated.
- Children 7 to 10 years old who did not have their full DTP/DTaP series (2-, 4-, 6-, and 15-month shots) need a Tdap shot.
- Children with an unknown or incomplete shot record or history before age 7 years need a Tdap shot.
- All adolescents with an up-to-date record need the Tdap shot at the 11-year well-child checkup/visit.
- Anyone older than 11 years who has not previously received DTaP or Tdap series needs the shot, when indicated.
- There's no minimum interval between Td and Tdap vaccines, meaning that if you for some reason had a Td (tetanus booster) in the last few years, you still need a Tdap now to protect against whooping cough. No 5- to 10-year interval is required between the shot.

- Pregnant moms are now recommended to have a Tdap shot during each and every pregnancy, sometime during the final trimester.
- Vaccine protection for pertussis, tetanus, and diphtheria fades with time, so adults need a booster shot. Experts recommend that adults receive a Td booster every 10 years and substitute a Tdap vaccine for one of the boosters.
- *Getting vaccinated with Tdap is especially important for adults who are around infants—new parents, grandparents, babysitters, nannies, and health care professionals.*

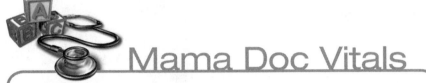

Mama Doc Vitals

Note: Although whooping cough got its name because of the characteristic loud, whooping sound that adults make when they have the infection, whooping cough in babies and children often just looks like a typical cold for the first 2 weeks. Trouble is, it can manifest into its other nickname—"the 100-day cough."

Tip: Babies are at biggest risk of serious or life-ending complications from whooping cough. They are most vulnerable between birth and 2 months of age but can have complications, including breathing cessation, up to about 6 months of age. Cocoon your newborn; surround her with family and friends all vaccinated against whooping cough.

Fact: In the 1990s, the vaccine used to protect against whooping cough changed from a whole-cell vaccine to an acellular vaccine. This change decreased side effects from the shot. However, we're learning with time that the acellular vaccine many not trigger similar levels of immunity; the protection the newer shot gives doesn't last as long.

Measles in America

If you're like many parents, you've probably heard more about the risks of the measles, mumps, rubella (MMR) shot than the risk of measles, mumps, or rubella infection. Reality is, the science is astoundingly clear: the risk of side effects from the MMR vaccine is far less than the risk of the illness itself.

Measles is a serious illness. Measles causes rash, runny nose, and fever, but can sometimes also lead to infections causing seizures, pneumonia, brain damage, and death. In 2011, 42% of children younger than 5 years who got measles here in the United States were hospitalized. Even with the best care, 1 to 3 out of every 1,000 children who get measles will die from the disease.

WendySueSwanson MD @SeattleMamaDoc

Infants 6-11 months of age who are traveling internationally should get MMR shot. Then next dose at 12 mo of age per CDC schedule. #measles

Shots do, of course, have side effects, but the vast majority of side effects are minor. Soreness at the injection site and an elevated temperature tend to be the most common side effects. Moderate side effects, including seizure from fever, a drop in blood cell count (platelets), or joint aches, are even less common. Life-threatening allergic reactions occur rarely (around one in 1 million doses), and more serious side effects often happen so infrequently that it's difficult to know if vaccines even caused them.

I've never cared for a child with measles. But I know many pediatricians who have. In the past couple of years, one of my friends let me know that her son contracted measles during a Midwest outbreak from an unvaccinated child. He was too young to be immunized (younger than 12 months). Even writing that sentence puts prickles down my back.

My friend, pediatrician Natasha Burgert, MD, FAAP, wrote the following after diagnosing measles during a 2011 outbreak in Kansas City:

I had never seen measles before. In fact, my practice partner 36 years my senior had never seen measles. As the vaccine-preventable disease continued to spread within my community, I could not help but think the majority of providers in Kansas City had also never seen a child with the classic rash.

The probability of the diagnosis being missed was very high, simply due to lack of experience with this childhood disease.

My suspicions of this phenomenon began to come true as stories began to emerge.

The outbreak in the Kansas City area had well over a dozen cases that likely weren't included in the total number of measles diagnoses, suggests Dr Burgert.

As the news of more measles cases began to surface, the reality of our small planet became glaringly evident. We believe that an infected traveler from Europe brought measles to my quiet, unassuming, flyover state. One person's choice—a half a world away—was affecting my families in KC. The responsibility we have as a global community to protect ourselves, and each other, from vaccine-preventable disease now weighs heavy on our community's hearts.

Not long before this book went to print, there was a huge outbreak of measles unfolding in Wales. More than 800 cases of measles had been confirmed in a small area during spring 2013, with one death reported in a 25-year-old. According to national immunization uptake data, Wales is known to have low vaccine update for MMR—only 82% of teens have had 2 doses of MMR by age 16. At the time of the outbreak, many experts theorized that the large number of unimmunized people in the population allowed for such dramatic spread of disease.

Mumps causes fever, headache, pain in muscles, and swollen glands. It can lead to deafness, infection in the brain, painful swelling of the testicles (or ovaries), and rarely can leave children sterile. Fortunately, the number of cases of mumps decreased dramatically in the United States following the introduction of the mumps vaccine in 1967, from an estimated 100,000 to 200,000 to fewer than 300 cases annually. In the United States, since 2001, an average of 265 mumps cases has been reported each year.

Recently, however, there has been an increase in the number of mumps cases reported. For example, in 2006, more than 6,000 cases of mumps were reported across the nation due to an outbreak.

Rubella causes a rash and arthritis (mostly in women, not girls) and fever. In children, rubella is usually mild with only a few noticeable symptoms—things like a fever or sore throat. Adults get more moderate infection symptoms that cause headaches, pinkeye, and overall discomfort for 1 to 5 days before the rash appears. The big reason to get all children immunized: if a woman gets rubella when she is pregnant, she can miscarry the baby, or the baby could be born with serious birth defects.

Vaccinated children are protected from infections but also protect their future playmates by preventing the spread of rubella to pregnant moms.

The MMR injection has never had thimerosal (a mercury-containing preservative) as an ingredient...*ever.* That myth lingers and remains rampant. And the myth confuses and scares parents. The shot, like any vaccine, does carry risk. The MMR vaccine causes fever in more than 10% of children (often 7 to 12 days after the shot as the immune system appropriately responds), a rash in 5% of children, and some swelling in the glands in cheeks or neck in about 1 out of 75 children. More serious problems include seizure caused by a fever in 1 out of every 3,000 doses given, pain in joints in adults, and low blood platelets—the cells that cause your blood to clot—in 1 out of every 30,000 doses given.

WendySueSwanson MD @SeattleMamaDoc

MMR vaccine causes thrombocytopenia in 1 of 30,000 doses. Rare risk. Benefit of protection/not getting measles (!!) still outweighs risk.

When you detail side effects, it all can sound a little scary, but the bottom line is that countless studies find that getting the MMR vaccine is much safer than getting measles, mumps, or rubella infection. And the MMR vaccine is remarkably effective; more than 99% of patients who get the series at 1 year and 4 years of age are immune to measles. These immunizations save not only our children's lives but also those in our community too sick or too young to be immunized.

58

Do You Believe in Vaccines?

A few years back, I wrote 33 pediatricians an e-mail asking what they would say, while in line for coffee, to the parent of a newborn when asked if they "believe in vaccines." I wrote the e-mail not as a gimmick or a way to frame the issue of vaccine hesitancy but because this happened to me while in line for coffee.

WendySueSwanson MD @SeattleMamaDoc

Just wrote 33 pediatricians an email w one question: "Given 2 minutes to represent vaccine while in line for coffee, what would you say?"

Thing is, this *happens* to me. Often. People have asked me repeatedly if I believe in vaccines.

This question comes up as families learn more about health online. This question comes up as parents remain concerned about vaccine safety, the number of vaccines given, and the safety record for immunizations given.

We start to give immunizations on a child's day of birth (hepatitis B) and at nearly every wellness visit in the first 2 years of a child's life. Clearly, this is a big part of our experience while in the examination room with our pediatrician or nurse practitioner.

When a new father asked me this question in line for coffee while carrying his newborn, I told him what I thought. But after I left the coffee line I immediately started to worry that I hadn't done a good job. I then ruminated about my response for 24+ hours before I wrote a group of colleagues. How do we talk with parents we don't know, outside of the examination room, to help them understand why we feel so strongly about protecting children with vaccines? How do we compassionately yet passionately display what we've learned about vaccines in preventing disease?

I'm not a believer in scripts. I'm not attempting to suggest there is a single 2-minute segment for every family about immunization safety that will help. I wanted to hear what these expert pediatricians would say to get a sense of their collective insight. I want you to see it, as well. I want to be really good at my job as a pediatrician when helping families understand the science, evidence, and emotion behind raising healthy kids and preventing illness with vaccines.

I also really want families to understand why pediatricians work so hard to vaccinate children. I don't want to increase the divide between those parents who are worried or skeptical of the possible harms of immunization and those parents, doctors, and experts who believe in the benefits. Rather, I want to regain our similarities.

We are all so similar.

We all want to do what is right for our children. That's why everyone is so passionate about their take on vaccines. Simply stated, we all care immensely.

This passion and commitment was confirmed when I wrote doctors from all parts of the United States. I got more than 20 responses. That's a pretty good response rate.

I've arranged these pediatricians' thoughts based on how I experienced their comments.

- Emotional
- Evidenced
- Experienced

These thoughts are not mutually exclusive; you'll hear evidence in the emotional comments, experience in the evidenced ones, and emotion in the experienced ones.

Part 1: Emotion

It isn't just parents who are emotional about vaccines. Pediatricians (and scientists/ public health experts) are ultimately responsible for improving the way families understand immunizations. So this is weighty.

Most of these doctors wrote me about listening more than talking. But here's some of what they said.

—◦◦◦—

David Hill, MD, FAAP, a pediatrician in North Carolina, wrote

Boy, is this an issue on all of our minds! For me, this question has particular poignancy, as we all watched our partner's (a pediatrician) 22-year-old daughter die of H1N1 last year. To see her facedown on a ventilator, bloated and pale, and then to have a parent tell me, as one did last week, "Everyone knows the flu vaccine causes just as much disease as it prevents."

Gulp. His response to that parent's viewpoint?

Screaming seems inadequate.

—◦◦◦—

Ari Brown, MD, FAAP, is a pediatrician and author of the book *Baby 411*. She noted

The most effective [technique in talking with families] had nothing to do with science. It was all emotion (cue Jenny McCarthy's playbook here)—"I vaccinate myself and my family to protect them. I wouldn't do anything differently for your child."

Of course, nothing works 100% of the time, but I can honestly say that this message does work more effectively than all the rest, and yes, it takes less than 2 minutes.

—◦◦◦—

Natasha Burgert, MD, FAAP, a general pediatrician in Kansas City, MO, helped define the scope.

The decision to vaccinate or not to vaccinate is far too important to make based on a "best seller" or a TV special.

—◦◦◦—

Ed Marcuse, MD, MPH, FAAP, a pediatrician and professor of pediatrics at the University of Washington, said

I don't have an elevator speech. My objective is not to sell immunization but to prompt [discussing] the decision not to vaccinate.

—◦◦◦—

Evelyn Hsu, MD, a gastroenterologist now specializing in liver disease and transplants, said

It's so nuts. I like to describe vaccines as invisible helmets for our children. Given the choice, it is the best way to protect them from unexpected danger. I've read about and have witnessed the power of the vaccine against hepatitis B, one of the most infectious viruses out there. Trust me, there are plenty of hepatitis B viremic [contagious] kids out there—most [who] can't yet be treated, and we just cross our fingers and hope that those around them are appropriately protected.

—◦◦◦—

—ᴄᴠᴠ꜀—

Pediatricians can feel frustrated with the ongoing task of discussing immunization and vaccine science in the examination room. It's certainly our job, but it can be arduous. It's difficult to have to defend science against anecdote. Emotion usually trumps the numbers. Which takes me back to something Dr Hill wrote:

It's said doctors crash three times as many airplanes as other private pilots. Why? Because we figure what we do is so hard anything else must be easy by comparison. Likewise it's the most educated parents who think they can skim the Internet for a half hour and say, "I've done some research." Whenever I hear this I'm dying to shout, "No, I've done tissue cultures, run gels, and crunched data. That's research! You read some [stuff] online, okay?" The immune system is complex enough for doctors. For a lay person, even a very smart one, it's like learning to fly an airliner. The principles seem simple enough, but what angle do you want the flaps at if you're landing in Denver with a little too much fuel on board in a 15-knot crosswind on the southeastern approach? The difference is we assume the pilot's interests are aligned with ours: to land safely. The educated public is skeptical of our motivations, so they figure maybe they'd better grab the stick and land this bird themselves.

—ᴄᴠᴠ꜀—

Skepticism runs deep in the public. I often hear claims that pediatricians give vaccines to make money. Not true, in any of my experience and teaching. And in many parts of the country, pediatric offices lose money giving shots (it's expensive to order, stock, refrigerate, give, and document vaccines). But anti-vaccination groups go to great lengths to confuse the public on the intention of pediatricians. With ads running in movie theaters warning against the risks of flu shots because of thimerosal, we are not safe from discussion about vaccines, even while chomping on popcorn before the movie. This is everywhere.

—ᴄᴠᴠ꜀—

Doctors think and worry about this out of the office, too. Dr Hsu described feeling worried and frustrated when children aren't protected.

[I feel] the same way I would feel when a non-helmeted kid gets hurt on his bike.

—ᴄᴠᴠ꜀—

—◊◊◊—

Pediatricians see children with vaccine-preventable illnesses as missed opportunities. It can be very emotional. And the memory of an ill child lingers. I also think pediatricians get emotional partly because of the daily reminders in their work.

—◊◊◊—

Doug Opel, MD, MPH, FAAP, a bioethicist, pediatrician, and father, said

I just came from the hospital where we have several kids hospitalized with whooping cough, some so severe they can't even breath on their own. To me it's just so tragic seeing these babies motionless on the hospital bed with a tube down their throat, IVs everywhere. I have my own kids and just can't imagine what it'd be like to see them like that…struggling to breathe and in pain.

—◊◊◊—

Paul Offit, MD, FAAP, an infectious disease and vaccine expert, author, and director of the Vaccine Education Center at the Children's Hospital of Philadelphia, wrote

I would make the case that a choice not to get vaccines is not a risk-free choice. Rather, it's a choice to take a different and far more serious risk.

—◊◊◊—

Bryan Vartabedian, MD, a pediatric gastroenterologist and blogger, said

Two minutes. Tight territory for 2 generations of work spent eliminating deadly childhood illnesses. Almost too short a time to change an opinion. I'm going to take a lesson from the antivax warriors…call it advocacy for those who can't speak for themselves:

Your daughter has the privilege of being born into the world at a time when deadly communicable diseases of infancy are effectively unheard of. Diseases that at one time could have left this precious baby blind, deaf, and mentally disabled are now found only in textbooks.…As this baby's mother, you have the sole responsibility to protect her and keep her out of harm's way. Your baby can't make the decision. You have to do it for her.

—◊◊◊—

———ᴥᴥᴥ———

Matthew Kronman, MD, FAAP, a pediatrician and infectious disease specialist, said

I've been mulling this over. In fact, 2 nights ago it kept me up a little bit (which nothing does, other than my daughter's cries).

He continued with a list of evidence (which is on page 242). But also said the following:

Vaccines DO have some rare side effects. The chances, on an individual level, of having one of the truly significant side effects are FAR LESS than the chances of having a car accident while driving to the office to discuss these things. They are FAR LESS than the odds of being struck by lightning in your lifetime. Bad things happen in this world, and the odds of having one of those bad things happen to you are HIGHER than the odds of a bad thing happening from a vaccine. So the very process of existence in our society carries more risk.

———ᴥᴥᴥ———

Alanna Levine, MD, FAAP, a pediatrician in New York, wrote

One of my "family activities" this weekend was taking my kindergartner to a birthday party where I was approached by one of the moms in his class. She had been to my Web site and saw that I was emphatically pro-vaccine and asked me about it because she "gave her kids the vaccines in the hospital and then not again until 15 months so she would only have to give them the bare minimum." When I asked her what she was afraid of, she replied, "It just seems like too much. I breastfed, I let my kids crawl on the floor and eat dirt. I figured that was enough." She seemed very proud of her decision and I, of course, could not resist the urge to talk her ear off for a good 20 minutes (I far exceeded the 2 minutes you proposed in your question!). I proudly explained to her that I too breastfed my kids and didn't shield them from dirt, but that I also vaccinated them and that is what I recommend to my patients. Today I got an e-mail from her about the class Thanksgiving party and at the end she added a PS that read, "Thank you also for your honesty and candor about vaccinations. Living where we do it must be so hard to get your point across. And yes, in the end I guess we are lucky nothing happened to our kids."

———ᴥᴥᴥ———

—◦◦◦—

Dr Burgert also said

I do believe in vaccines. What I believe in even more, however, is my responsibility as a pediatrician to partner with a family to make this decision easier. I know choosing to vaccinate is a very emotional subject and is hotly debated in many families. But, this is not a war.

—◦◦◦—

Part 2: Evidence

As I said, I'm not a believer in scripts. I'm not attempting to suggest there is a single 2-minute segment for every family that will help. Part of the reason I started writing about my experience as a mom and pediatrician is that in practice it became evident that when I told families what I knew and learned in training, they listened. When I told them what I did for my own children and how I felt, they made decisions. Telling my story seemed essential.

Rather than talk to you about numbers, reaction rates, and the absence of thimerosal in all childhood vaccines (except multidose flu shots for children older than 3 years), these comments focus on the evidence that helps physicians discuss immunizations with families.

There is no evidence that an alternative vaccine schedule is safer. There is no evidence that an unimmunized child is safer. And there's a lot of history to prove to us that vaccines save lives. But here's what my friends and colleagues wrote.

—◦◦◦—

Gayle Smith, MD, FAAP, a general pediatrician in Richmond, VA, said it best.

I'd say how much I wished pediatricians were better "rock stars" with our message of prevention so we could be more effective in the media limelight. I'd speak my own willingness to touch the hearts of the families I care for, to carry the bag of fear and worry for them, perhaps lessening their load a bit.

—◦◦◦—

If you're interested in reading studies about autism and vaccines, the safety of thimerosal, or neurologic outcomes after immunizations, look at "Vaccine Safety: Examine the Evidence" (see "Mama Doc Vitals" on page 248). I often discuss the last study in this list with families. Lots and lots of evidence. But in my experience in the office, data are ultimately not very helpful for families who are fearful of vaccines.

—◦◦◦—

—◦◦◦—

Ellen Lipstein, MD, FAAP, a general academic pediatrician at Cincinnati Children's, said

For me, and I hope for my patients, vaccines aren't about beliefs but about evidence. In all the decisions we make for the people we love, we have to balance the evidence of risks with the evidence of benefits. For me, there is no doubt that vaccines are highly beneficial for the person [who] receives them, their family members, and the general community. They are not without risks, but the risks are very small compared to the risks of not vaccinating.

—◦◦◦—

Flaura Winston, MD, PhD, FAAP, a pediatrician and founder and co-scientific director, Center for Injury Research and Prevention, the Children's Hospital of Philadelphia, said

I concur with the "motivational interviewing" approach for patient counseling. It is NOT one-size-fits-all persuasive discussions. Rather, it moves the patient/family to positive behavior change through a partnership. One of many recent reviews can be found in the December 2005 issue of Archives of Pediatrics & Adolescent Medicine *(Volume 159).*

—◦◦◦—

Dr Lipstein again

In working with families who are vaccine hesitant, I think a valuable option would be to take a page from the shared decision-making literature. Specifically, we need better resources that visually depict risks. Traditionally (perhaps not surprisingly, nearly all this work is in adult medicine), tools that help individuals determine their values and risk preferences have been limited to situations where there is nearly absolute clinical equipoise, 2 equally good (or bad) medical options. Think prostate and breast cancer screening and treatment. However, we know that individuals struggle with decisions that the medical community thinks are relatively straightforward and not situations of equipoise. Taking the lessons from these other settings may help us design resources that facilitate parent understanding, clinical discussions, and choices that everyone can live with.

—◦◦◦—

—◦◦◦—

Dr Opel also said

Given that parents consistently report that their child's provider is the most important influence in their immunization decision-making, we really should have a good idea of what we should say to parents. For instance, studies of doctor-parent communication since the 1960s have found that parents better adhere to recommended treatments and are more satisfied with their visit if they felt that their concerns were understood. A provider's interpersonal sensitivity and empathy have also been linked to improved outcomes.

Dr Opel referenced a Centers for Disease Control and Prevention (CDC) handout as a great resource for pediatricians working on improving their skills in communicating about immunizations and added

We are currently conducting a study in which we are videotaping well-child visits to do just this. The hope is that by directly observing what providers actually say and how parents respond, and then linking these provider communication behaviors over time to the child's immunization status, we can know which communication techniques are linked with improved immunization. A start, I suppose.

—◦◦◦—

Denise Shushan, MD, a pediatrician working in the Seattle area, said

I do spend some time with some families who are concerned about MMR/autism, in particular detailing that the research of Dr Wakefield has been thoroughly and repeatedly discredited, as well as informing families that his original intent was to discredit the existing MMR vaccine because he was hoping to sell his own version of the MMR. Most parents are quite receptive and surprised—I think it reminds those people who are intent on believing the "Big Pharma is fooling everyone just to make billions hawking their dangerous vaccines" meme that the supposed saint whose research linked autism and MMR vaccination was motivated by something far less altruistic than they might otherwise believe.

—◦◦◦—

Dr Brown noted

The percentage of cautious parents has risen and fallen depending on the news cycle.

—◦◦◦—

—∿∿∿—

So, what do you say to the cautious parents? Much of it is not talking, but listening. Studies have shown that in low-concern settings, people look to the experts for advice. In high-concern settings, people look to the empathetic listener, not the expert.

—∿∿∿—

Doug Diekema, MD, FAAP, a bioethicist and emergency department pediatrician, said

First, I make people aware that they may be putting other children at risk by not vaccinating their own children—that almost every school has someone who has cancer or an immune deficiency and who would be placed at risk if they came in contact with an unvaccinated child who had pertussis or measles or chickenpox.

Second, I think we can recognize parents' concerns about vaccines and share our own concerns about children who are unvaccinated. In the past 6 months, pertussis has killed 2 infants in Washington and more than 10 in California. Those are real children killed by a real disease that can be prevented by vaccines. In just 2 states, 12 deaths in 6 months. Even the wildest scare tactics of the anti-vaccine crowd can't match that in terms of devastation.

—∿∿∿—

Dr Kronman said

Some people cannot be immunized, and immunizing your child will protect them too. At times children are too young to receive vaccines, and others who have cancer or other immunocompromising conditions cannot be vaccinated. Vaccinating your child will protect her, but it will also protect your aging father on chemotherapy. It is good for your child AND for society.

Life expectancy has risen over the last century by 20 years or more, and much of that is due to NOT CATCHING AND DYING FROM DISEASES PREVENTABLE BY VACCINES.

—∿∿∿—

Dr Brown pointed out

One study in Pediatrics *in 2006 categorized parents into 4 groups: believers, relaxed, cautious, and unconvinced. The "cautious" group is the key group that we should focus our attention to. Believers and relaxed parents believe in vaccinations and they believe in their health care provider to head them in the right direction....Unconvinced parents will never change their minds about vaccinations no matter how much time and effort you spend talking and educating them.*

—∿∿∿—

———◈◈◈———

Melissa Arca, MD, FAAP, a general pediatrician, said

Do I believe in vaccines? Absolutely. Are they completely risk free? No, but in reality nothing is really risk free. It essentially all comes down to the risk-versus-benefit ratio. The benefit of vaccines far outweighs any rare or perhaps theoretical risk associated with them. After all, [parents] only want to do what is right by their children and to not cause harm.

———◈◈◈———

Dr Marcuse added

I know full well that while science does not have all the answers, it is the best way to get reliable information. But I know there is good and bad science and [it] can be hard to sort out.

———◈◈◈———

Dr Offit wrote

Diseases like whooping cough, mumps, and measles are again starting to rear their heads, causing children to suffer and die. And although vaccines, like all medicines, can cause side effects, the ones you hear about (like autism, allergies, learning disorders, multiple sclerosis, diabetes, among others) aren't caused by vaccines. So the risks that most people fear aren't real risks.

———◈◈◈———

Dr Marcuse concluded by saying

I refer [parents] to unbiased sources of good science-based information. At the top of my list is www.NNii.org because I can say it accepts no funds from vaccine manufacturers or the government and its only mission is to provide sound information to help parents make well-informed choices.

———◈◈◈———

Part 3: Experience

Helping families make decisions about their child's health takes training, expertise, and experience. The training is standardized (medical school, residency, fellowship) and the expertise confirmed by passing board examinations and maintaining yearly continuing medical education. But the experience piece is ultimately unique for each physician. With each day in clinical care, patients teach, instruct, and shape how we understand wellness and illness. Through individual experiences with patients, physicians ultimately become who they are in the examination room. In medicine, despite the huge push to standardize everything from centralized phone calls to how much (or little) time we get with patients, individual doctors will fortunately remain unique. As patients, we still get to enjoy our physicians as people helping us through illness and injury.

A physician who cares for me repeatedly reminds me how much I learn from being a patient in health care. She's entirely instructive for me as a patient and as a physician; her bedside manner astounds. I believe she's just very good at her job, partly because she's uniquely experienced. I believe her experience being a nurse for many years before becoming a doctor really colors how she provides care—she gets it.

I've been thinking about immunizations, reading comments on my blog, writing about vaccines, and witnessing my patients' responses. I've received many e-mails. Immunizations and discussions about the schedule are a huge part of my clinic days.

Of course, experiences in clinical care (and living on planet Earth) shape how all pediatricians discuss and listen to families when discussing immunizations. Here's more of what my friends and colleagues said about their experiences discussing vaccine schedules and vaccine safety.

Dr Kronman, a pediatrician and infectious disease expert, said

We don't see these diseases anymore. I work at a premier tertiary/quarternary care facility for children. I have seen children die of influenza (seasonal, H1N1), pneumococcus, meningococcus, the late sequelae [side effects] of measles, pertussis; I have seen Hib meningitis, tetanus, severe debilitating outcomes with varicella, cervical cancer caused by HPV, and severe rotavirus. This list goes on. But most people haven't seen these things anymore. People don't have to panic about their children in the summer becoming permanently paralyzed from polio because we don't see it anymore. And the reason? Vaccines.

Dr Burgert said

In other parts of the world where I have briefly practiced medicine, I have seen the faces of grieving families whose children have died from vaccine-preventable diseases. Those families did not have the equal opportunity that you have for your family.

Natalie Vogel, MD, FAAP, a general pediatrician in Northern California, said

With patients in clinic, and when thinking about immunizations, I come back to thinking about how hesitancy is about a person's personal perception of risk. Understanding risk is so complicated and personal! It pits fact and epidemiology

("science") right up against emotion. My sense of risk is very different from the next person's. Addressing that sense is crucial in a discussion of vaccines with a tentative family.

———

One comment, from Alison Buttenheim, PhD, MBA, a researcher working with Dr Winston, furthered what Dr Vogel mentioned. Dr Buttenheim discusses her experience and research focused on improving pediatricians' skill in discussing immunizations.

These clinical interventions are likely to be marginal. We recently completed 23 in-depth interviews with parents in a high-SES [socioeconomic status] urban neighborhood, most of whom I would classify as hesitant but ultimately adherent (lots of requests for spaced schedules). One clear take-away from this qualitative research is that parents know what they want to do long before the first well-child visit. Among the more hesitant parents in our sample, the choice of a pediatric practice was based in part in finding a provider who would accommodate an alternative schedule. I think we need to focus our research on parental decision processes outside of the [doctor's] office and how they are shaped by media, peers, etc. Attention to cognitive heuristics and biases (such as how we interpret risk and look for confirming but not disconfirming evidence) should reveal promising opportunities for communications and policy interventions.

———

Dr Shushan added

When I've talked about this with parents in the [ED], I always begin by acknowledging the profound mistrust that has developed in the community between vaccine-making companies, physicians, and families. I also acknowledge that, while I think that the vast majority of cases of serious events that occur near vaccine administration times are coincidental, there may be a subset of kids in whom the immune reaction generated by vaccine administration stimulates some preexisting propensity for medical badness (obviously, I don't say it that way, but my brain is fried after working all night). In my opinion, our job is to research this issue to try and determine if there is such a subset of kids, and if so, to figure out how to identify those kids. We trust most parents on their gut feelings on so many other occasions. Yet, as a profession, we are quite dismissive (which seems arrogant to families) of parents who describe a deterioration in their child after immunizations. I don't think that helps our cause any.

———

Dr Kronman emphasized

I HAVE AND WILL CONTINUE TO PROVIDE ALL OF THESE VACCINES FOR MY OWN CHILDREN. In 2010, I had to go to health center #2 and stand in line for 4 hours last year to get the H1N1 vaccine because [our pediatrician's office] didn't have it yet. And standing in that line was certainly a risky proposition in south Philly. But it was the right thing to do. Simply put, immunizing your child protects her.

Dr Opel said

I find myself in your scenario a lot…maybe not with complete strangers, but certainly with new-parent family members right before an immunization visit who call me for my "opinion" and from neighbors who stop me walking my dog to ask me where I stand on giving my patients and my own kids the H1N1 vaccine. I usually follow some version of ask-tell-ask. That is, I don't give them a one-liner, "You should do X or do Y," from the get-go. Instead, I let them talk first: "Well, let me first hear how you are thinking this through? What are fears? What have you read? What have others told you?" That kind of thing….It's easier [for parents] because I think it is far more manageable to correct misinformation in 2 minutes than it is to summarize the breadth of the pros and cons of immunizations.

Dr Hill wrote

I'd like to think it helps that I vaccinate my own 3 children and myself. Sometimes, when I mention this, it does. But sometimes I just get that look that says, "So you drank the Kool-Aid, huh?" What we're facing with vaccines, I fear, is but one symptom of a medical reimbursement system everyone knows is crooked. We pay enormous sums for procedures and a pittance for preventive care, so why should anyone think what we do has value? People read every day about psychiatrists who collect huge sums speaking for PHRMA, orthopedists who implant the hardware they've invested in rather than what's been proven best, about laminectomies, meniscal shaving, and arterial stent insertions doctors perform with no evidence whatsoever they work better than placebo. We sold the public hormone replacement therapy, COX-2 inhibitors, and Baycol. We know what we're saying can be trusted, but the public often feels they can't tell.

—⟞⟋⟋⟋⟍—

Dr Hill also said this, which I think I've repeated to about a half-dozen people since.

I like the quote from the "All Things Considered" piece on physicians as PHRMA speakers, noting that not only do we teach doctors to think critically in medical school, we teach them that we've taught them to think critically. For this reason, doctors assume they are impervious to the noncritical-thinking–based persuasion used by drug reps.

—⟞⟋⟋⟋⟍—

Maybe we really need to step back in pediatrics and reevaluate how we discuss vaccines. Authority and expertise, per se, may not be the right context in which to discuss this. In my practice, I talk about the experiences I've had with vaccine-preventable illness but also the experience of how it feels being a mom when intervening with shots.

—⟞⟋⟋⟋⟍—

Dr Arca said

Parents, I believe, just want to know that we [as pediatricians] "get it"; we understand where they are coming from. We do; we are parents too and have made these same decisions.

—⟞⟋⟋⟋⟍—

Dr Smith said

I'm one of those people who remembers infantile paralysis. That's what they called polio when I was a young child. I do believe in vaccines. I remember my great grandmother saying, "Don't go play over on Shiloh Street because that's where the little boy died of polio," and I grew up in Pittsburgh where the initial polio vaccine trials took place. Mothers in my neighborhood had the opportunity to be a part of history, to vaccinate their child with something that might save a life. In the beginning, nobody knew for sure that the vaccine would work without unacceptable side effects. They only knew that too many children died or were left paralyzed by this horrible virus. My great grandmother, who wasn't afraid of anything, embodied the visceral fear that this germ could claim the life of her grandchild. That memory left its indelible mark.

I do believe in using the body's natural, God-given ability to save itself from disease. Vaccines give us a way to make immunity without paying the huge price of illness, maybe even death, to get that protection. Yes, I believe in vaccines, and I am grateful for them…just like my great grandmother.

—⟞⟋⟋⟋⟍—

Continuing this discussion about immunizations is essential.

Mama Doc Vitals

Where to Go Online to Read About Immunizations

- For accessible scientific information, look at the Children's Hospital of Philadelphia Vaccine Education Center (www.vaccine.chop.edu), with constantly updated information on the science and safety of vaccines from world-leading pediatric experts.

- National Network for Immunization Information: www.NNii.org.

- The American Academy of Pediatrics (AAP) Web site designed for parents, www.HealthyChildren.org, is easy to read, has great information, and is backed by a force of 60,000 pediatricians making up the AAP.

- Every Child By Two, a foundation to help families understand the need for timely (up-to-date) immunizations, has a Web site with videos and resources on getting your child's shots if you can't pay for them: http://bit.ly/mdm-ECBT.

- Don't ever hesitate to read about vaccines at the CDC Web site. It has comprehensive information for patients and families: http://bit.ly/mdm-CDCvaccines.

- "Vaccine Safety: Examine the Evidence": http://bit.ly/mdm-VaccineSafety.

- My blog! Go to www.seattlemamadoc.com and search under the tag "vaccines."

Pediatricians' Conditional Comfort With Alternative Vaccine Schedules

You may know what your friends think of alternative vaccine schedules, but what about pediatricians? There's little we know about the safety of alternative schedules, but that being said, physicians have differing comfort when families request vaccine delays.

I spoke with my friend Doug Opel, MD, MPH, FAAP, about his 2011 study about pediatricians and alternative vaccine schedules. He's a pediatrician, dad to 2, and bioethicist trying to improve understanding about why parents hesitate or delay vaccinations. I learned a lot while we spoke. There is great wisdom in what he said that extends far past what he learned in the study.

Dr Opel is one of those genuinely authentic, kind people. He's the kind who never speaks too loudly or too soon. The kind of person you meet and wonder, gosh, if only I could be a fly on the wall when he's making decisions for his kids or decisions for his life or decisions for his patients—you know you'd be better off. He's the kind of guy you want on your softball team or around when you really get worried about your child. He's remarkably thoughtful, so there is no wonder this study illuminated some helpful observations.

Dr Opel and his colleagues conducted a survey of Washington pediatricians to find out how often they were being asked about alternative vaccine schedules and how doctors felt about it. Not surprisingly, 77% of pediatricians reported that they are regularly being asked to use an alternative vaccine schedule. And in general, the majority of pediatricians (61%) stated they have become "comfortable" with alternative schedules, but only for particular vaccines. Meaning that although pediatricians are OK with parents' request to delay some vaccines (hepatitis B or polio), they are not comfortable waiting on others (diphtheria, tetanus, acellular pertussis [DTaP], *Haemophilus influenzae* type b [Hib], or pneumococcal conjugate [PCV]). The reason, Dr Opel suggests, is that pediatricians are unwilling to leave kids unprotected from potentially devastating diseases that still circulate in our communities.

Dr Opel lends insight to the culture of concern about vaccine safety, how the changing health care environment has shaped how we ask questions in the examination room, and how the concern about autism and vaccines is simply emblematic of concerns about vaccine safety in general.

Some pediatricians refuse to see families who don't immunize. Most often, the reason is protection of vulnerable populations of patients in the waiting or examination rooms. Babies too young to be immunized or children on chronic medications that don't allow them to be vaccinated are at risk if an infected child (who could have been immunized) comes into the office with a vaccine-preventable disease.

Although some pediatricians draw those lines to protect vulnerable patients, most of us spend a great deal of our time in clinic discussing vaccine benefits and risks and working with families who request alternative schedules. And the majority of us (in Washington) are comfortable, at least in part, with alternative vaccine schedules. I don't think we've been left a choice with the requests from our patients. Yet this comfort only goes so far. As Dr Opel states, it's a conditional comfort. It depends on which vaccine a family is asking to delay.

The hope from this study (in Dr Opel's words) is that parents will know that "…pediatricians really are here to work with you and to help you make these decisions." He also hopes that this will help spawn more research on alternative schedule safety because, as he explains, "If parents are asking for these schedules frequently, we ought to know how safe they are."

Here's the majority of the conversation I had with Dr Opel.

Why do the study?

Dr Opel: Our collective clinical experience was that we were seeing more kids where parents were requesting an alternative schedule. We wanted to find out about Washington state pediatricians' preferences and comfort with parents' requests for alternative vaccine schedules. We also know from other data in the state, parents are opting out of required school entry immunizations more now than they have in the past. We also felt it would be important to document whether [parents asking about alternative schedules] is actually true. I think there are ramifications to the results. If parents are asking about alternative schedules frequently, we should know about their safety and effectiveness.

We wanted to get a sense of the collective experience of pediatricians. The more and more requests we see to deviate from the vaccine schedule of the Centers for Disease Control and Prevention (CDC), the more we wondered about how pediatricians were responding.

What did you find?

Dr Opel: Deviations from the recommended schedule are occurring, and pediatricians are responding that they are fairly comfortable with them. Overall, 77% of pediatricians reported that parents sometimes or frequently requested alternative schedules. Recent reports have shown on the national level that a significant number of parents are requesting this in other parts of the country. So the study confirmed our hypothesis that it's a regular occurrence. Furthermore, 61% of pediatricians said they were comfortable using an alternative schedule if requested by a parent.

In the study, you wrote, "Parental acceptance of childhood immunizations is waning." Why do you think that's true?

Dr Opel: I think it's got a complex and multifactorial root cause to issue of vaccine hesitancy. Three things contribute to it most.

1. **The changing infectious disease environment.** We don't have a lot of the diseases we used to have around (no smallpox, no diphtheria, no polio). Without them around, there is just a natural tendency for us to not be concerned about these or at least perceive them as less severe.

2. **Changing health care environment.** My father was a pediatrician, and when he counseled families regarding recommendations, there was very little resistance to the recommendations he gave. Since that time (20–30 years), there has been a rise in consumerism that has affected health care, where parents feel empowered to take charge of their health care. Generally this is a good thing, but consequences are that parents feel compelled to not accept recommendations that their providers give them. And that might include vaccine recommendations. There are also more easily recognized limits to what modern medicine and science can do. Increasingly, science has given us an amazing achievement in medicine, and that is vaccines. But increasingly the thought that modern medicine can't address many issues like substance abuse or obesity and that there are limits to easing the burden of chronic disease. Modern medicine is perceived as being less able to do this and less useful, and as we see these limitations, we feel that other places (like complementary and alternative medicine) can address these problems. And this feeds into how we accept traditional medical recommendations.

3. **How the media and the Internet have shaped this discussion.** With the rise in consumerism in medicine, there are messages for the consumer and they come from mass media. And unfortunately, those messages are anything but clear and straightforward. Rather, they are very conflicting and misleading. Parents have to navigate this. A lot of misinformation and controversy is propagated. That doesn't help hesitancy…in fact, it probably fuels it.

What will you do with the results?

Dr Opel: Well, if parents are asking about different schedules for immunizations, it has policy implications. Also, the more that parents request schedules outside the CDC schedule, the more we need to know about how pediatricians are talking about immunizations and the more we want those that set policy to think about these conversations.

Before Dr Sears' book, did parents ask about alternative schedules?

Dr Opel: I think the publishing of Dr Sears' book really popularized the notion that there are other schedules out there that are possible and that parents can request them from the child's pediatric provider. I think my sense is that it is a much more frequent request since his book, but in the study, we actually asked pediatricians if Dr Sears' book affected their willingness to use an alternative schedule. The majority said it didn't affect their willingness. Before Dr Sears' book, I'm sure that there were some parents who asked their provider if there was something different than what was recommended by the [CDC]. Now, there are parents who bring that book into my office, under their arms. His book has been widely read.

Do you think concerns about autism, which started in 1998 with false claims about measles, mumps, rubella (MMR) safety, affect parents today? Does it feed and breed safety concerns about known side effects of vaccines (like fever or rash)?

Dr Opel: The concern about autism and vaccines is emblematic of parental concerns about safety in general. Autism is devastating. It's every parents' fear that their child won't develop normally and be able to interact with them in the way they hope and dream of. Because it is such a feared outcome, it is a highest-level concern that most parents talk about when they talk about safety. But it doesn't mean that it is the only concern. You almost have to shed away that layer [concern about neurodevelopmental outcomes] and their concerns about very bad things, and then several other worries (rash or minimal side effect) can be addressed.

Pediatricians were more comfortable about waiting on certain vaccines; explain your thoughts about that.

Dr Opel: Pediatricians responded they were comfortable waiting on some but not on others; pediatricians had a conditional comfort with waiting. The 3 they weren't willing to delay or use an alternative schedule: DTaP, Hib, and PCV. We didn't ask them why they were less willing, but most pediatricians were unwilling to delay those. We thought the reasons that pediatricians were unwilling to delay was because these vaccines covered diseases that are still in active circulation (like pertussis that is currently endemic and we are suffering from an outbreak right now in Washington) and diseases that particularly have severe consequences for babies left unprotected, like meningitis. Also, there are severe consequences from the infections caused by the infections protected by Hib and PCV vaccines. These are things that can leave children devastated. I think this demonstrates reasonable judgment on the part of pediatricians. I think they are doing the best job they can when parents desire an alternative schedule. It really reflects this tension that providers are dealing with—the desire they want to respect a parent's decision but also an obligation to protect a child's health.

Pediatricians are standing firm on those vaccines that prevent diseases that children have a high risk of getting or life-threatening diseases and potentially being more flexible on other vaccines and yet being less rigid on the overall schedule.

What do you hope this study will do?

Dr Opel: On a parent level, I hope it shows to parents that pediatricians really are here to work with you and to help you make these decisions. And I hope it also shows parents that doctors are trying to do what is best for their child as well.

On a policy level, I hope this study moves the conversation toward better understanding of the safety of these alternative schedules and how effective they are, if at all, are they more or less effective than the recommended immunization schedule. If parents are asking for these schedules frequently, we ought to know how safe they are.

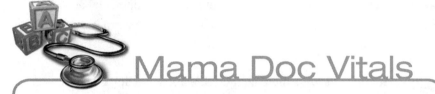

Mama Doc Vitals

Tip: There are no data to suggest any benefit for your child waiting to get a shot. A 3-year-old doesn't have less risk from the chickenpox shot than a 1-year-old. When children get delayed vaccines, they get all the same risks as they would have if they'd been immunized on time.

Pediatricians Who Refuse Families Who Don't Immunize

This question came up on during a chat on the *New York Times* "Ethicist" Web site.

What do you think about pediatricians who refuse patients who don't follow the [American Academy of Pediatrics (AAP)] schedule? Do you disagree with me? Would you be more comfortable seeing a pediatrician who refused those families who chose not to immunize to protect your children? Have you, or someone you know, ever been kicked out of a pediatrician's practice?

I'm a pediatrician (with a master's degree in bioethics) and mother to 2 boys. I will always keep my practice open to vaccine-hesitant families. However, the waiting room risk (unimmunized kids and risk to vulnerable populations, ie, infants, those too young for vaccines, and immunocompromised children) is a good one and the only compelling reason to close to patients who refuse immunizations, in my opinion.

But it's not a good-enough reason for me to send families away who have questions and hesitations about the AAP/Centers for Disease Control and Prevention schedule. All children deserve a pediatrician versed in immunization benefit/risk and an expert in conversation with their parents to foster insight and understanding. Frankly, if waiting room risk is the concern, there are ways to create separate waiting rooms for kids who are up to date and kids who are not.

Great thing is, only about 10% of families use alternative vaccine schedules. In a recent *Pediatrics* article, only 2% of families who used alternative schedules refused all vaccines altogether. So although this is a large issue in pediatrics and parenting, the majority of families do vaccinate on time or nearly on time. I don't want to lose sight of that.

I practice in Washington. We lead the nation in exemptions for vaccines (more than 10% of kids with exemptions vs only 2% nationally) and have recently put into place a law that requires families to consult with a health care provider prior to an exemption. It was designed to avoid exemptions out of convenience. This hopefully opens up opportunities for discussions with parents and pediatricians!

We all want the same thing—healthy children, healthy communities. Fostering conversation and diminishing a context of "war" or opposition about immunizations is an important step. In my experience, most parents end up immunizing their children over time, even when they start out as refusers. The group of full refusers is fairly small. So allowing all kids into my practice feels like a great opportunity.

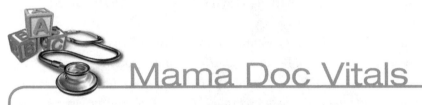

Mama Doc Vitals

Fact: Measles was transmitted to an unvaccinated child in a clinic waiting room during the 2008 California measles outbreak. This is one reason some pediatricians choose only to see children and families who immunize—they take the stand only because they want to protect their entire practice.

Most Parents Avoid Alternative
Vaccination Schedules

I see this as a glass half full, glass half empty issue. In 2011, a study was published in *Pediatrics* detailing research conducted in May 2010 about parents' preferences to use alternative vaccination schedules versus following the recommended Centers for Disease Control and Prevention (CDC) vaccination schedule. The majority of the media coverage focused on the finding that more than 10% of parents followed a schedule other than the one recommended by the CDC. Not perfect and not ideal from a public health standpoint. Yet, of course, the other way to see this is that nearly 90% of parents did follow the physician-recommended schedule. That's a pretty good success rate for doctors.

I saw this study as half full. As I read through the methods, results, and discussion, I took notes on the cover page. I actually made a little half-empty, half-full doodle. I couldn't help but think about the nearly 90% of families (87%) who followed the recommended schedule to protect their children and their communities. Clearly 87% is not 100% (I get that), and it leaves our communities and our children at risk, but I believe we can continue to improve trust with ongoing education.

Focusing on the group that does vaccinate their children on the schedule may be a good strategy to understanding where we can improve our communication about the benefits of vaccination. We often focus on the group that doesn't vaccinate, but we miss insight from those of us who do immunize our children on the schedule.

Details

The study was conducted on more than 2,000 respondents, where 771 families qualified by reporting having a child between 6 months and 6 years of age. They were asked if they followed the CDC schedule and then, if they didn't, they were asked to answer a series of closed-ended questions regarding the nitty-gritty of the schedule they used. Parents' age, gender, race/ethnicity, and level of education and family insurance were collected.

Glass Half Full Findings

- Only 2% of all the families interviewed refused all vaccines for their children. Two percent simply isn't much.
- Thirteen percent of parents reported following an alternative vaccination schedule, with most families stating they only refused certain vaccines (53% of them). This means that nearly 90% of parents reported following the CDC recommendations. That's nearly an A minus!
- Of the "alternative vaccinators," a large minority of parents reported having initially following the recommended schedule.
- Fifty-five percent of families that were on alternative schedules ended up giving all of the recommended vaccines but on a delayed schedule.
- Of the "alternative vaccinators," only 8% of that group followed a well-known alternative schedule such as that offered up by Dr Sears or Donald Miller, MD.
- Several families responded that they had worked with their child's physician "to develop the schedule." Fantastic. A true partnership between the patient and physician and one that is transparent and necessary for catch-up immunizations.

I imagine physicians screaming at me at this point, directing me to all of the issues with these findings and why they aren't necessarily positive. I'm not ignorant, but I still experience those findings as hopeful for our communities. Our job really may be activating those parents who do vaccinate and do follow the CDC schedule to share their stories and their "whys" behind protecting their children from harm with vaccines.

For me, the most concerning finding resided in a group that followed doctors' advice but doubted their own choice. Of the group that vaccinated their young children on the recommended CDC schedule, 28% reported that they felt the alternative schedule was actually safer. What? Oh no. This certainly serves as a wake-up call that we clearly aren't doing a good job explaining the benefits of the schedule. And we may not be checking back in with families after vaccinations. What I know in my heart is that parents want to do what is right for their children. This statistic challenges that parents feel reassured after vaccine visits. And it serves as a reminder for physicians everywhere.

Glass Half Empty Finding

- One in 5 parents who followed the recommended CDC schedule felt that delaying vaccines was safer than the CDC schedule they had used with their children. Unsettling. As the authors point out, this finding represents that 1 in 5 families may be "at risk" for changing to an alternative vaccination schedule. This would assume that housing doubt (about anything) would stop a parent from immunizing. In my experience, that's not exactly how parenting works. Sometimes, we do what is recommend by those we trust (our children's physician, a vaccinologist) because they are more expert than we are and understand more about the risks and benefits. And we sometimes remain concerned. I suspect this group represents that sentiment. And from my vantage point, late tonight after a long day in clinic, it seems like this is simply part of parenthood at times.

- Most families indicated that they came up with the new schedule themselves (41%) or took advice from a friend (15%) or family member.

- Twenty-two percent disagreed with the statement that the best vaccination schedule to follow was the one recommended by vaccination experts. Befuddling. If we don't let our national and world vaccine experts hold our trust, who should get it? I simply don't understand this. Remember, a recent study found that the far majority of parents trusted their child's pediatrician most when getting information about vaccine safety. Regardless, the 22% statistic confirms that we need to do more to explain how vaccine research is conducted and why it is best to immunize early to maximize protection for children.

- Eighty-six percent of families using the alternative schedule had refused the H1N1 vaccine for their children. Gasp.

- Seventy-six percent of families using the alternative schedule had refused the seasonal influenza vaccine for their children.

- The vaccines most commonly spaced out were the measles, mumps, rubella (45%) and the diphtheria, tetanus, acellular pertussis (43%). As many of you know, we have widely elevated circulating rates of pertussis (whooping cough) in the United States. An infant died in the county where I practice recently from whooping cough, while 2 other infants were hospitalized. Many studies have found that under-immunization in communities significantly increases the risk of contracting and spreading vaccine-preventable diseases. Further, for 2011, the Health District in Snohomish County (where I see patients in clinic) had 80 laboratory-confirmed or epidemiologically linked cases of pertussis reported. In contrast, for all of 2010, Snohomish County had only 25 cases, and for 2009, only 33 cases.

Because no vaccine is 100% effective, all of our children (and all of us) are dependent on an entire community being immunized to avoid vaccine-preventable diseases.

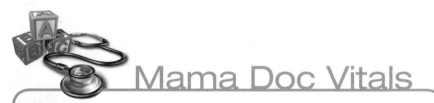

Mama Doc Vitals

Study: "Alternative Vaccination Schedule Preferences Among Parents of Young Children": http://bit.ly/mdm-AVSarticle

Scientific Opinion: "The Problem With Dr Bob's Alternative Vaccine Schedule": http://bit.ly/mdm-AVS

The Injustice of Immunization Interviews: Vaccines on the News

After Andrew Wakefield's study was retracted from the medical journal *The Lancet*, after he'd already lost his medical license, and after a series of investigative editorials were published that detailed his fraud in telling parents that measles, mumps, rubella (MMR) vaccine caused autism, he was invited to interview on *Good Morning America* (GMA). When this happened, an injustice occurred—for children, I mean. And it occurred inadvertently, I suspect.

I believe this injustice happens all the time when it comes to children's health and wellness. What the media covers really changes how we think and feel about protecting and parenting our children. The media's effort to inform and educate, just like that of physicians and nurses, social workers and ancillary staff, researchers and students, can get lost and misconstrued. ABC worked hard to inform us of the accusations against Dr Wakefield with a 2-minute introduction by Richard Besser, MD, FAAP, a pediatrician and medical editor/correspondent. Yet when the interview was over, I was left remembering the myth.

Studies show those who watch myths (even when paired with solutions) on TV can't sort out what data are the myth and what was fact.

Dr Wakefield interviewed on GMA with George Stephanopoulos, who later labeled the interview "combative." Mr Stephanopoulos was given a terribly difficult task: he was interviewing Wakefield on one of the most complex, emotional, and loaded quandaries of the last few decades—vaccine hesitancy and Wakefield's purport linking vaccines to autism. When Wakefield failed to deny any allegations and failed to discuss the significant research that refutes his own work, Mr Stephanopoulos had to defend science. Alone. George Stephanopoulos isn't gaining popularity with the anti-vaccine crowd and even some who doubt what Dr Wakefield claims. Yet ultimately, the 7-minute interview with Stephanopoulos and Wakefield simply stirs the pot. I trust it had huge viewership. I worry that this is, in part, why it was done.

We need to discuss immunizations in the context of which decisions about immunizations are made. At this point, interviewing Wakefield alone does not serve children or our public well. His myth and legacy regain power with each second he's on the news. We need to have discussions about immunizations that reflect the fear that has arrived on parents' doorsteps because of Wakefield's work. We needed a general pediatrician, a parent of immunized children, and a vaccine expert in the interview too. Having Dr Besser in the interview can be a great start. We need voices of reason. We need to frame issues surrounding immunizations truthfully. Although Dr Wakefield made claims that he didn't want others to stop immunizing for diseases like whooping cough (pertussis), his work is at the core of hesitancy in the United States for all vaccines. George Stephanopoulos needed to make that point clear.

Although Wakefield now defends and talks about one vaccine (MMR), he fueled millions of parents to distrust all of them.

In the office, when parents who are hesitant about immunizations talk about their worry, they often point to Wakefield's claim as one big reason. However, as the years unfold from the uncovering of Dr Wakefield's fraud in the *British Medical Journal,* I hear less worry from families about his purport that MMR vaccine causes autism. However, this interview on GMA is illustrative of Wakefield's ongoing power. Seven minutes alone in front of millions is power.

In Dr Besser's introduction, there were some micro-interviews (sound bites) of Paul Offit, MD, FAAP (vaccine expert and pediatrician), and Seth Mnookin (author of a new book, *The Panic Virus).* Neither were given the time and exposure Wakefield received. What we learned from Dr Offit and Mr Mnookin about immunizations could easily be forgotten by the time the interview with Wakefield was over.

Continuing to wage a war between those who want to immunize and those who don't isn't working. Parents are increasingly more confused, not more informed, after these interviews. Although some bloggers are declaring vaccine hesitancy dead since the information in *BMJ* on Wakefield's fraud was published, I think we're far from seeing the end of vaccine hesitancy. Distrust in our physicians and nurses only increases when stories and interviews occur in this fashion. I believe I will be listening to and helping families concerned about immunizations for the rest of my clinical pediatric career.

> *Continuing to wage a war between those who want to immunize and those who don't isn't working.*

Let's change how we report and discuss issues around vaccine hesitancy and the "controversy" in vaccine research. We need to realign patients with the physicians and nurse practitioners who care for our children. Our children deserve better than to force parents to do "research" online about immunizations, as Dr Wakefield suggests.

Dr Besser has extensive experience caring for children in practice and an impressive history of leadership in academia and at the Centers for Disease Control and Prevention. He did a wonderful job summing up the state of where we are on vaccine hesitancy in this country. But Dr Besser's introductory segment wasn't enough. We leave the interview with Wakefield and go back to our cereal thinking about the "war" over vaccines. The interview this morning accelerates vaccine hesitancy in the United States rather than illuminating what science holds. The interview was a near fistfight, demonstrating our differences as parents rather than our similarities.

We must regain our similarities; we all want what is best for our children. Pediatricians and researchers are parents too.

> *It can take only seconds to create a myth. It can take decades to rebuild the truth and refute the myth.*

George Stephanopoulos had an opinion as the interview began; he stated he had read Dr Wakefield's book and made it clear that he didn't believe what Dr Wakefield was saying when responding to statements. I agree with the commentary on the ABC blog that he had seemingly made his decision prior to the start of the interview. This is sensible; science really goes against what Andrew Wakefield has claimed. Dozens of large studies have refuted the claims Wakefield made long ago. His research has been retracted by *The Lancet*. His coauthors have backed away from their words and affiliations. *We already knew all this.*

It can take only seconds to create a myth. It can take decades to rebuild the truth and refute the myth. That's where we find ourselves today.

The editorial in the *BMJ* uncomfortably put Wakefield back into the spotlight. His message, although rebuked, gained more power today. Regardless of the "truth" held in science that vaccines have not been found to cause autism, Wakefield "won" the interview today. Hands down. Arm wrestled George to the floor. His message is memorable. And he puts the onus again on our shoulders as parents and physicians.

We are left remembering Dr Wakefield's name, the title of his book, and his take. He instructed, "My recommendation for parents is to read; there is extensive information out there." He alienates us from the pediatricians, family doctors, and nurse practitioners who care for our children. Should we imply he doesn't want us to trust physicians or scientists? He leaves the work up to parents. But this controversy sells.

Viewership is the economy of television. If you're going to get people to watch, putting Dr Wakefield in the hot seat is a great way to start. But that's where the injustice occurs. Instead of clarifying, we are left more confused. As in politics, fear and controversy rage on, it seems.

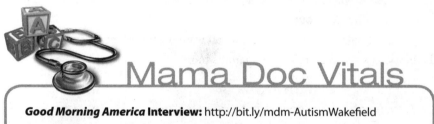

Mama Doc Vitals

Good Morning America Interview: http://bit.ly/mdm-AutismWakefield

Brian Deer's Article: "Wakefield's Article Linking MMR Vaccine and Autism Was Fraudulent": http://bit.ly/mdm-AutismDeer

Fact: MMR vaccine has never contained the preservative thimerosal.

Pile on the Paperwork: Vaccine Exemption

I'm happy about a new pile of paperwork piling up. New laws around the country require vaccine exemption to be signed by medical doctors. I'm not living under a rock; I understand that some feel these new bills requiring signatures for vaccine exemption are heavy handed.

I wholeheartedly disagree.

Vaccine exemption laws require families to talk with a health care worker about the risks when exempting from immunizations. It turns out that Washington lags in its vaccination rates compared with national averages. In the last 10 years, there has been a doubling in the number of students with exemptions for vaccinations in our schools. The biggest reason may be a convenience

Imagine this...

You're a busy parent whose child is about to start kindergarten or sixth grade. The records you have for her immunizations are incomplete. You didn't keep the shot record book and like me and everyone else, your paperwork isn't filed perfectly. You're pretty sure your child is up to date. You're standing at registration at the school. You've been waiting in line and your left heel hurts. Come to think of it, your head hurts too. Your daughter just tugged on your pant leg; she's hungry. Quickly, when you realize you've got an incomplete record, you call your daughter's doctor's office while still in line. No one picks up when you call and you're put in a queue waiting to talk with someone in medical records. *You have a choice:* Would you rather just sign your name, exempting your child from vaccines? Or would you rather go on a hunt for the records to ensure your child truly is up to date? Sure, the answer for most any parent is clear.

You sign your name.

See? It doesn't make any sense to have an exemption, with weighty consequences, be so easily misapplied. We're busy and tired and disorganized and have overwhelming demands. These exemptions, where children potentially miss shots they may need, puts our entire community at risk. Further, during a breakout of chickenpox or measles or pertussis, the Department of Health would have to contact your family and track down the records to know if you're at risk or if others are at risk because of an unimmunized child. We know that unimmunized children are more likely to get and spread vaccine-preventable illness. It's expensive to track inconsistent (exempted but immunized, exempted and not immunized) records down in an outbreak. And it's becoming more common.

factor. The state suggests that 95% of exemptions are not for a medical reason but one for convenience. Seems like you'd never opt out of immunizations for convenience, putting your child or another child at risk. Right? But then think about how nuts your life is, how chaotic it is to raise children, and work, and pay bills, and....

Realities About Vaccine Exemptions

Many children everywhere rely on the community to be well immunized to stay healthy. Many suggest we need 90% of a community to be immunized to prevent an outbreak of illness. Studies show that children in schools with higher exemption rates (lower immunization rates, likely) have higher levels of disease. And as I said, we know unimmunized children are more likely to get and spread vaccine-preventable illnesses. We want to protect, or cocoon, our most vulnerable (young infants, patients with immune dysfunction, or those children on chemotherapy who can't get vaccines). Maybe you're one of the parents who didn't want to opt out, but out of convenience and/or pant-tugging-snack-needing-headache-relieving necessity while in line, you did. In this case, if your child wasn't truly up to date (immunization guidelines change yearly), there would be little incentive to go out of your way to ensure she received needed immunizations.

This convenience factor and need for "community immunity" was the reason for the bill. The bill isn't about forcing or battling with families who are hesitant or opting out of immunizations for religious reasons or concerns about vaccine safety. This isn't about selling vaccines. The bill works to counter families who opted out accidentally or out of convenience. The bill works to increase public education about vaccines. The bill works to get more children the immunizations they need. It's to protect our community and our most vulnerable children. If families want to opt out, they still can opt out, but they will have to have a conversation with a health care worker prior. Think of this as an insurance plan for all children, demanding we all make choices with great intention rather than just convenience.

That's where the pile of paperwork comes in. Physicians will now need to sign off on exemptions. I will happily sign these papers for families if they decide to opt out or exempt from immunizations. But I'll do so in person, in clinic, once we've discussed risks.

This bill for paperwork allows parents to access information about vaccines from physicians and nurses, the people parents say they trust most on vaccine safety.

Some Statistics About Exemptions in the United States

The national average exemption rate is estimated to be less than 2%, most recently published as a median exemption rate of 1.5%. That means less than 2% of families in the United States refuse all vaccines.

- States allowing for the option of a philosophical exemption often have conditions.
- Of those 19 states, most have various conditions to getting a philosophical exemption above just a parent signature.
- Seven states require you to submit a written statement for exempting (Louisiana, Maine, Michigan, Ohio, Oklahoma, Pennsylvania, Wisconsin).
- Three states require the forms to be notarized or to be a signed affidavit (Arkansas, Minnesota, Texas).
- Four states require some kind of educational component on risks/benefits of immunizations (Arizona, Arkansas, Vermont, Washington).
- Seven states require direct involvement from the local or state health department (Arkansas, Idaho, Missouri [child care only] North Dakota, Texas, Vermont, Washington).
- Three states require renewals (Maine is ever year; Texas is every 2 years; Vermont is every year).

Some of the more recent states "expanding" their laws to allow philosophical exemptions are the ones with the most conditions. For example, Texas "expanded" its laws in 2003 but requires that you request the state health department send you the form, you sign on the form that you've read and understand the attached immunization materials (supplied by the state department), you have the form notarized, and the form expires after 2 years—at which point you start all over if you want to continue the exemption.

In most states in the United States it is up to families, in consultation with health care workers, if they immunize their children. Families will first have access to health information about vaccines/immunization and the risks they incur when exempting prior to entering school.

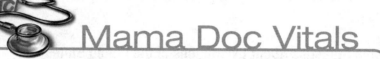

Mama Doc Vitals

Tip: Exemptions allowed vary by state, and data on how many children are exempted in your child's school are collected by the state. Numbers may be difficult to find. Ask your school or call the county health department and ask for an online link with the numbers.

Keep the Book

Data collected here in the United States determine that carrying an immunization record for your child can improve his health by increasing the likelihood of staying up to date on shots. When my boys got their H1N1 shots, I didn't bring their immunization record books. I was all hyped up and excited about getting them for protection, and because the shots were given outside the regular pediatrician's office because of the rush to immunize the community, I forgot the shot book. I was given a little card at the time but didn't transfer the dates into their official books. When back in the office, I had to discuss and review the records with staff until we ultimately completed their medical record. Not a big deal, but it wasted precious time for the staff in the clinic.

A study published in 2010 brings merit to keeping and carrying your child's immunization record or book, particularly if you don't follow the recommended American Academy of Pediatrics schedule or your child has received immunizations from multiple different physician offices. The study found that if you carried and kept a shot record for your child, you could increase the odds by 62% that your child would be truly up to date. Often, parents feel their child is up to date when in reality, he's not. This is often because of updated recommendations; a messy, incomplete record; or new boosters children need. Carrying and keeping the records yourself can clear up confusion, dispel doubt, and sometimes avoid unnecessary redos to immunizations. Most children don't have the fortune of seeing the same pediatrician from birth to age 18, so carrying a portable copy of their immunizations may reduce error and confusion. Keep the book, an easy (maybe?) way to advocate for great and perfect health care for your child.

Staying on Top of Immunizations

Here's how I see it.

- Let's be honest; kids get lots of shots. This is an incredible fortune in the world of trying to avoid threatening, preventable disease. Help ensure your kids get the right doses at the right time. To my count, including yearly flu shots, children can have up to 50 inoculations before they head off to college. Even if you don't want your child to get all the shots when recommended…keep the book!

- Always keep an immunization card (book) for your child in your home; don't rely on the pediatrician's office. Cards are often handed out in the birthing hospital. If you've lost the card, ask your pediatrician for a new one at the next visit. Have the medical assistant fill it out with the data they have and double-check your own copies.

- Sign up for a medical portal or "MyChart" at your doctor's office if it has an electronic medical record. That way you'll always have access to your children's medical record to print out when needed for school, sports teams, or travel. In the age of digital medical records, the paper card can be a reliable way to track your child's immunizations, particularly if your child has been to more than one pediatric clinic. Don't yet rely on technology to do this for you. Errors unfortunately do occur. Keep the book.

- Keep the book where you keep those important papers, like the lien on your car, the mortgage, that favorite rookie baseball card. When your now toddler applies to medical school, it will be easy to prove she's had her hepatitis B series!

- If you forget the card at a visit, bring it in the next time your child sees the doctor. It's not only at well-child checkups that we confirm the record, add to your book, or update immunizations.

If there is no record of a shot, pediatricians will always err on the side of caution and redo a dose of the immunization. This is safe and can ensure your child is protected against illness, but speaking from experience, it never feels great to give an immunization that may not be needed. By keeping the book, you may avoid excess or repeat doses of an immunization by confirming it's already been done.

Keep the book, then. Yes, please. I'm tucking ours in between the medical school loans and the mortgage. Prized possessions indeed.

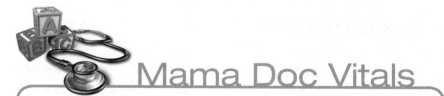

Mama Doc Vitals

Tip: Download the American Academy of Pediatrics HealthyChildren.org Child Health Tracker app for tracking your child's shots: http://bit.ly/mdm-HealthTracker.

65

Fear of Needles

Vaccine hesitancy comes in all flavors. It's not always concerns about safety that causes children, teens, and parents to hesitate or even refuse vaccines. Sometimes it's about pain. Or simply discomfort. Or anxiety. It's perfectly natural, of course, to have a fear of needles. It's rare that a child enjoys the pain of an injection (although those kids, even at young ages, are out there).

Sometimes the fear and anxiety of needles really can manifest itself as a sincere phobia. In those cases, the fear is so overwhelming that it changes family decision-making around vaccinations and leaves children unprotected. It can torture parents when they have to scoop their kids up from under the chair. And parents get embarrassed when their child/teen becomes combative with shots. Sometimes they avoid coming back to clinic simply to avoid the conflict. Makes sense in a hectic world.

In clinic, I took care of a teen soon after she'd had a terrible experience with influenza (the "flu"), and it's changed how I care for my patients. She was a high school student with asthma. Because of her asthma, her doctor had recommended a flu shot. Even though doctors recommend flu shots for all children between 6 months and 18 years, we work very hard to get high-risk patients protected. Children and teens with asthma are more likely to have severe pneumonia after contracting influenza. We worry about children who wheeze and have asthma (even mild asthma) because it can land them in the hospital or cause a life-threatening illness.

Most parents of children with asthma get flu shots yearly, early in the season. But not all.

When I saw the girl in clinic she was exhausted and stressed, confused and scared. Through the course of her influenza illness, she had missed 2 weeks of school and lost more than 15 pounds. She was still coughing a few weeks later. I looked back to the chart note visit prior to her infection, in which her pediatrician had recommended the flu shot. *"She'd declined,"* it said.

"Why?" I asked.

She stated that she was terrified of needles. Because of her persistent asthma, she wasn't allowed to get the nasal spray flu vaccination (wheezing is a contraindication), so the shot was her only option. "Had you told the doctor your reason for saying 'No?'" I asked.

"Yup," she said. But no plan of action was made to support her.

So here's the thing: we know that fear and anxiety about injections worsen when a parent is scared too. When I asked her mom if she was scared, she nodded. Often, the declination for vaccination prolongs if parents are scared of the injection. Again, it makes sense. But after the experience of the illness, she and her mom were very motivated to figure out how to get the shot next year.

During the injection, parental demeanor clearly affects the child's pain behaviors. Excessive parental reassurance, criticism, or apology seems to increase distress, whereas humor and distraction tend to decrease distress.

Tips to Support Your Child When Fear of Needles Arises

- Don't make promises for "no shots" any time you are going to the clinic. You never know what plan will be recommended and what shots you've missed. If you make and break that promise, trust is broken. Don't joke about the doctor or nurse giving a shot as punishment either. No single shot is ever given to make a child uncomfortable; don't create that myth, as it sets your child up to believe that the doctor may harm her.
- Fear of needles is real. Validate your child when he states he is terrified. And then talk directly with the clinician about ways to support your child during the shots.
- Consider using an antianxiety medication (something like Ativan, Valium, or Xanax) when true needle phobia is present. I've worked with a pediatric psychiatrist for numerous patients in my clinic to develop a plan for using medication and other anxiety-breakers to support them getting recommended care.
- Consider using a numbing cream (something like EMLA or vapocoolant spray) to numb the skin prior to vaccination. You'll need a prescription from your clinician to do so, but often the cream provides a bit of comfort and a sense of control and boosts confidence for anxious or fearful children/teens.
- Consider deep breathing and other behavioral modifications, including distraction at the time of injections, to support your child. Consider seeing a behavioral health clinician as well.

- Consider the "cough trick." I offer the cough trick to all of my patients and teens nervous about shots. Studies (and reports from my patients) confirm it works brilliantly!

Mama Doc Vitals

Study: "Pain Reduction During Pediatric Immunizations: Evidence-Based Review and Recommendations": http://bit.ly/mdm-PainPrep

Tip: Studies find that excessive reassurance, apologies, or criticism from parents about shots increases a child's distress when getting shots. Be honest; don't say it won't hurt (it likely will). Do your best to chill out during shots. Offer distraction for your children and incentives to do it quickly and get back to play!

Tip: The "cough trick" can be practiced before shot visits so your child or teen can be a pro. Have your child practice a forceful, fake cough. Then have your child designate which arm in which she wants the shot. She then can determine that on the count of 3 (for example), the medical assistant or nurse injects the vaccine. Right when the nurse injects (on 3), your child does another fake, forceful cough. Children report less pain, as do their parents and nurses, when using this technique.

Fact: You can get skin-numbing creams at the pharmacy over the counter, or you can ask your doctor to prescribe one in advance. Don't overpromise a miracle; keep in mind that most needles inject into the muscle or into deeper layers of the skin, so pain will not disappear entirely.

66

People Are Dying From the Flu

Influenza virus causes "the flu." It's a crummy cold that spreads easily, causing high fever, body aches, runny nose, terrible cough, and rarely, vomiting and diarrhea too. The flu isn't the "stomach flu." It's deadlier than that. It's more dangerous for babies and young children and for the elderly. It's also particularly dangerous for those with asthma, diabetes, and neurologic or immune problems. *This is a bit of a plea:* People continue to die from the flu every year and there are ways we can potentially save others' lives.

The Bad News

Flu usually peaks in February or March. Different strains become the dominant strain of flu that moves around the United States. In 2013, for example, the most common strain circulating was called H3N2—it's known to cause more serious disease. At its peak, more than 80% of our states were reporting widespread circulating levels of flu. Where I lived at the time in Washington, 6 people had died, one of them a child younger than 12. A healthy 17-year-old in Minnesota had also died the week before. Flu is not just your "common cold"; it can be far worse. Eighteen children have already died this season. As of November 2012, we didn't even have half of our population with a flu shot. The goal to protect us all is 90%.

I've never had a family in clinic get influenza illness and then refuse the flu shot the following year. They come in early and often for their shots. It can be that bad of an illness.

The Good News

We have a vaccine for the virus that causes the flu. The flu shot and FluMist nasal spray are catered to what strains we expect each year. You'll be protected against the flu somewhere from 10 to 14 days after getting it. Go out now and protect yourself and your family. By getting a shot, you protect yourself, your children, and all those more vulnerable in our community who are unable to get the shot (infants younger than 6 months, those on chemotherapy, or those with contraindications to the shot).

Debunking 5 Myths About the Flu

- **The flu shot doesn't cause the flu.** The shot is an entirely dead virus—
  it's impossible for it to replicate in your body and cause infection. The
  nasal spray is a very weakened strain (imagine a sprinter without legs or a
  bumblebee without wings) that is unable to replicate in the lungs to cause
  disease. The most common side effects after the shot or nasal spray are
  fatigue, low-grade fever, and runny nose (from the nasal spray).

- **You may feel like you "don't get the flu."** Well, chances are that you do
  or you might. Research shows that anywhere from 5% to 20% of all adults
  get influenza *every year.* Anywhere from 10% to 40% of all children get
  it annually as well. Sometimes it's just a mild infection; sometimes it's far
  worse. You may not know you've had it unless a clinician tests you.

- **The flu shot doesn't work.** It does work, but like every shot, it's imperfect.
  It is possible for someone to still get the flu after a flu shot, but the infection
  is far less severe when he or she has had the shot. Each year the flu shot can
  change in effectiveness due to differing strains that are included in the shot
  and that may circulate in your community. You need a flu shot every year
  because the influenza virus mutates while moving around the globe.

- **I'm healthy, so I don't need a flu shot.** We're lucky that we're healthy, but
  don't let that fool you. Healthy children and adults die from the flu every
  year. Often about half of the children who die from influenza (usually a
  couple hundred each season) are healthy infants and children. About 30,000
  people die every year from flu in the United States. The flu shot you get now
  can help protect you.

- **If you don't "do" flu shots but you now have a child, you must change.**
  Your children, particularly those younger than 4 years, and those infants
  too young to get a shot (younger than 6 months) are utterly dependent on
  you getting a flu shot so you don't bring influenza home to them.

Why a Flu Shot Every Year?

People ask me every year why you have to get an annual flu shot. Here's why.

We know that influenza virus changes each and every year. It mutates and
changes its shape to kind of survive. Well, we don't want it to, and it takes the
efforts of people all over the world. There are more than 100 different centers
in 100 different countries that are gradually, all year long, tracking what types

of influenza viruses patients are having. They report back to 5 major centers in Australia, London, Atlanta, Japan, and China, and they look at what types of infections are inhabiting humans and causing disease.

Then, as we get close to flu season this time of year, these centers decide what makes up the annual vaccine. Each year since the 1980s there have been 3 strains of influenza in the shot or nasal spray, 2 types of influenza A virus and one type of influenza B. Now this year we have one that's very similar to the old H1N1, another type of influenza A, and a new influenza B. This is coming out of data from around the world of the flu that's moving across the globe.

You need it annually because you add on to the immunity that you gained each and every year you've been exposed to influenza-like viruses and influenza shots. Now kids older than 9 years only need a dose of the shot or the spray; for kids younger than 9, it depends on how many shots they've had in the past. Talk to your pediatrician or family practitioner about what kind of flu shot your child can get, but that's a little bit about the science of how it comes to be and which 3 strains get in each year.

67

Varicella Vaccine: It Works

I don't diagnose chickenpox often. I've seen patients with chickenpox only a handful of times since I started medical school in 1998. Auspiciously, there simply haven't been many children to serve as my teachers. Varicella virus causes chickenpox...*and there's a vaccine for that.* So, like smallpox or polio, I've been forced to learn a lot about chickenpox in textbooks. My strongest professor in the chickenpox department is my own memory; I had varicella between the ages of 5 and 6 years. It was the one week of my childhood when I remember being really babied—my mom gave me a small gift or craft every day while I was home from school. I got to watch TV on the couch. I was a completely TV-starved child because of my mom's rules, so I must have looked pretty awful. But it wasn't so bad and I was lucky. I was a healthy 5-year-old girl who had a case of chickenpox that was "run of the mill": lots of spots, lots of itching, and a week of fever and feeling crummy. Then poof, I scabbed over and got better. The only remaining trace (besides the virus that may live in my nerves) is the scar on my forehead. You can see it in photos.

The big trouble with chickenpox is that you can't predict which child will have a serious complication—a brain infection, an overgrowth of flesh-eating bacteria in the sores, or life-threatening pneumonia.

While I was finishing up college, the varicella vaccination was introduced in the United States. At that time, more than 150 people died every year from chickenpox, and more than 11,000 people were hospitalized annually. This created a huge economic toll (from missed work to health care costs).

So my apparent lack of clinical opportunity with chickenpox reflects reality. A recent study published in *Pediatrics* found that over the last 12 years, *there has been a 97% reduction in deaths from chickenpox in children and adolescents younger than 20 years.* There has been an 88% reduction in chickenpox deaths overall (kids plus adults). These are staggering statistics.

Varicella and Varicella Vaccine in the United States

- Prior to the mid-1990s, varicella caused hundreds of deaths every single year. It caused thousands more hospitalizations.
- Since 1995, we've been vaccinating children between 12 and 18 months of age against varicella (chickenpox). Some children can't receive the vaccine (those with, for example, suppressed immune systems, a history of recent bone marrow transplant, or cancer), so they are protected by those vaccinated.
- Between 1997 and 2007, only 77 total people died from chickenpox.
- Between 1997 and 2007, the rate of those vaccinated against chickenpox increased from 27% to 90%!
- In 2002, we started to do a booster dose for varicella at 4 to 6 years of age to increase protection against chickenpox. We have been catching up all other children with another dose, and now when children enter kindergarten, every child should have 2 doses total. The reason: research has found that 1 dose of the vaccine is 85% effective in preventing all varicella, but with 2 doses, effectiveness rises to 97% to 100%.
- Most of the 77 deaths occurred in patients "without apparent contraindication to vaccination" who didn't receive the shot. Therefore, those deaths were potentially preventable. Major missed opportunity...
- **The vaccine works.** Of the 77 total deaths since 1997, only 2 deaths were in children who had received 1 dose of the varicella shot. Both of those children were on steroid therapy (suppressing their immune system), and one of the children had cancer.

This tells us that we're living in a wonderful era in which few die from chickenpox disease and complications. We've created a safer environment. If your child is born now, gets the varicella vaccine, and has no other immune-related medical problems, the likelihood of dying from chickenpox disease is nearing zero. Further, through the combination of your own immunization and the protection of the "herd" of vaccinated children around you, you're even better protected too.

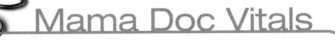

Mama Doc Vitals

Study: "Near Elimination of Varicella Deaths in the US After Implementation of the Vaccination Program": http://bit.ly/mdm-ChickenpoxShot

Tip: Your baby is well protected against chickenpox during infancy thanks to maternal antibodies that passed through during pregnancy. However, at 1 year of age, immunity is wearing off. Get your child her chickenpox shot at 1 year of age. If your child gets exposed to chickenpox as a toddler, she can go right in to see the doctor and get the second varicella vaccine dose immediately to protect her. If she gets the second dose early and prior to her fourth birthday, she won't need another dose before kindergarten.

Fact: Chickenpox has nothing to do with poultry. Chickens don't cause or spread chickenpox infections.

68

Hepatitis A: A Vaccine for That

The Centers for Disease Control and Prevention declared an outbreak of hepatitis A in June 2013 that affected more than 150 people in 10 states. The source of the outbreak stemmed from organic frozen berries that were sold at Costco stores. It's typical for Americans to get hepatitis A from contaminated food.

The amazing thing about the outbreak: there were very few children affected (only 11). None of the children who became ill had been vaccinated with hepatitis A vaccine.

Our children are well protected!

In the United States, hepatitis A typically spreads through contaminated food handled by someone with the infection. Rates of hepatitis A infection tops 5,000 to 10,000 cases annually in the United States, while they are far higher in the developing world because city water sources can get contaminated. Hepatitis A vaccine is recommended before international travel.

The absolute lack of vaccinated children with infections from this outbreak is logical and potentially illustrative.

Thing is, there's a vaccine that provides long-term immunity against hepatitis A. We now immunize all children against hepatitis A after their first birthday. We started immunizing all children against hepatitis A after 2006. Prior to that, children living in communities with high rates of hepatitis A infection received the shots.

Hepatitis A is spread through contaminated food. Hepatitis A symptoms tend to be more mild in children when compared with adults. However, hepatitis A is a *hepatitis*—meaning the viral infection causes inflammation of the liver. When infected with hepatitis A, children can have jaundice (yellowing of the skin and eyes), vomiting, diarrhea, and nausea. Rarely, the infection can cause hospitalization. However, I vividly remember admitting a child with hepatitis A to the hospital while a resident physician. She was sick, vomiting, and bright yellow....

If you want to protect yourself from hepatitis A, the best thing to do is be vaccinated. Fortunately, children are far better protected during these outbreaks, as we immunize all children in the United States. At the next checkup, ensure your children are up to date, especially if they were born before 2006, as the hepatitis A 1-year-old shot wasn't routine prior to that.

The Kids Are Lucky: The Hepatitis A Shot

- Hepatitis A vaccine is given to all children starting at 1 year of age. We give the first dose at the 12-month-old well-child appointment and the second dose at 18 months of age. Children need 6 months between the 2 doses. More than 95% of children who get their shots are protected against getting hepatitis A infection.

- All children are recommended to get catch-up doses of hepatitis A vaccine if they haven't had it. Prior to 2006, children only received hepatitis A vaccine if they were living in a city or county with higher rates of infection. If your children were born before 2006, ensure they have received the catch-up for this 2-shot series throughout the last few years.

- Hepatitis A vaccine is a very successful vaccine with few serious side effects. Pain at the injection site is the most common side effect, followed by headache in 5% to 10% of people. The benefit of hepatitis A vaccinations far outweighs the small risks of the shot. The vaccine has been given to millions of people without serious side effects.

- Consider hepatitis A vaccination if you're traveling to Asia, Central or South America, the Mediterranean Basin, Southern Europe, the Middle East, Mexico, and the Caribbean. It's recommended that every traveler get hepatitis A vaccine 1 month prior to international travel. But even if it is just 2 weeks prior to your trip, go get hepatitis A vaccine if you haven't. Evidence finds that immunity (as measured by antibodies in your blood) can rise days after the first vaccination against hepatitis A and may protect you on a trip in the upcoming 2 weeks. If you're traveling in the next couple of weeks, call a travel clinic, as there are other ways to protect yourself against hepatitis A infection during travel via immune globulins.

- The Vaccine Education Center at the Children's Hospital of Philadelphia explains travel risk as follows: "Because hepatitis A virus is present in the stools of people who are infected, countries or cities with low standards for the handling and disposal of sewage have an enormous problem with hepatitis A virus infections. The problem is that the virus quickly enters the water supply and contaminates anything that comes in contact with the water. It is probably not unrealistic to think about many developing countries as having a thin layer of hepatitis A virus that covers anything that you could put into your mouth."

  YUCK!

Chickenpox Parties

In April 2013, a Seattle mom advertised on an online parenting community that both of her children had chickenpox and invited (non-vaccinated) children over for exposure. It turns out that people are still having chickenpox parties. This was no April Fools' joke.

> Date: Mon Apr 1, 2013 1:19 pm
>
> I no longer immunize for the pox, and I have two children with it now. For those of you who are hoping your child gets pox and thus it's [sic] lifelong immunity – cone [sic] on over for coffee! Lol.
>
> No, really… ;)

Part of this makes my head spin. I just don't get it, despite having had many families in my practice decline, hesitate, or delay the chickenpox shot. I don't think parents know what virus they are dealing with. After I posted this invitation on Twitter, I had physicians all over the country sharing stories (some included here).

Chickenpox can cause serious infection complications and, rarely, can be lethal. Before the vaccine was approved and put into use in 1995, hundreds of children and adults died in this country every year from chickenpox and thousands were hospitalized. Although most young children get chickenpox and recover (only left with pox or scars), some children develop life-threatening secondary infections. Some children develop severe pneumonia (1 in 1,000 children), some develop brain infections, and some develop flesh-eating bacterial infections in their scabs that can even be fatal.

There is a safe, highly effective vaccine for chickenpox: varicella vaccine.

After I saw the pox party invite this afternoon, I became slightly enraged. I mean, there are *numerous* children and adults in our community immunosuppressed and/or on chemotherapy who could develop life-ending complications if exposed to varicella. And some families are intentionally exposing their children to a potentially harmful infection. After 2 doses of the chickenpox (varicella) vaccine, 99% of patients are immune to chickenpox. Although some children can get chickenpox once vaccinated, they typically only have a few pox and do not develop severe side effects or die.

The pox party just shows me how much work we have to do to build trust in vaccines and vaccine safety. My boys have had 2 doses each of the varicella vaccine. I'm thrilled they are protected and unlikely to ever get chickenpox or spread it to a community member who could be more at risk. They likely won't get shingles either.

More Chickenpox Facts and Stats

- Varicella shots hurt on injection (children tell me it really stings). We give the shot twice, once at 1 year of age and once at 4 years of age. The shot can commonly cause arm soreness and low-grade fever. In fewer than 5% of children, a small rash develops, often around the site of the shot. That's a good sign that the immune system is being triggered to fight off future infections. The rash that can develop after the shot is not contagious.
- Live chickenpox is super-contagious. I love this stat from the Children's Hospital of Philadelphia Vaccine Education Center: take 100 people, put them in a room with one infected person with chickenpox, and let them talk for a couple hours. Over that time, 85 of the 99 people will get chickenpox.
- Children with chickenpox are contagious for a day or 2 before the pox appear. That means your child with a low-grade fever and runny nose could go to school for a couple days, expose hundreds, and then present back at home as having chickenpox a couple days later when the pox develop.
- The varicella vaccine is a live-virus vaccine that induces protection in a similar way as vaccines against measles, mumps, and rubella. Therefore, because the vaccine creates copies (around 20) of the virus to stimulate immunity, our bodies respond like we've been infected; protection is likely to be lifelong. A study published in *Pediatrics* found that after even one dose of the shot, immunity was long lasting: "This study confirmed that varicella vaccine is effective at preventing chicken pox, with no waning noted over a 14-year period." Ongoing surveillance of lifelong immunity in vaccinated children and adults will continue through our lifetimes.

- Shingles is a reawakening of varicella infection (painful blisters that follow the path of a nerve), often in those older than 45 years or those who have weakened immune systems. People who have had the varicella shot (versus the infection) are far less likely to get shingles.
- A teenager or adult who has never had chickenpox should get the vaccine.
- If your child is exposed to chickenpox, call your pediatrician, and you can come in for the first or second shot if your child hasn't yet had it.
- Pregnant women who get varicella can pass on risks to unborn babies. One out of every 50 women who gets chickenpox during pregnancy will have a child with a birth defect.

WendySueSwanson MD @SeattleMamaDoc

Seattle mom posts info for chickenpox party the same day a study finds long-lasting protection from the shot: bit.ly/XndLup

70

Don't Make Promises: Yearly Immunization Update

New immunization recommendations come out every February. They're released to assist parents and clinicians in keeping all children up to date and protected from life-threatening infections. The update reflects new science and discoveries while improving the schedule of vaccines due to outbreaks of infection or improved understanding of how to better protect children amid a potential resurgence.

This is relevant to every parent: Every year, the rules for what children need which shots when can change. Just when we think all of our children are up to date, new science evolves that potentially changes their immunization status.

We have to do our best to avoid making false promises to children about "not needing a shot" when they go to see the doctor. Just when we do, we find that our child is due for a necessary booster or missed vaccine. Commonly, children are missing the last shot in a series of immunizations (eg, to protect children and teens from human papillomavirus [HPV], they need 3 total shots; children haven't had the second chickenpox shot). In my opinion, the promises broken break trust with our children and amp fear around going to the doctor.

Don't make a promise you can't keep. Probably something your mother told you. I'm not pointing my finger, but I often tell this to families in anticipation of a pediatrician's visit too. Do your best not to promise "no shots" prior to a visit. Although you may think your child is up to date on shots, she may not be. Or the pediatrician may order a blood study (seems like a shot to a child) or injection that you're not anticipating. And then we're all in a sticky situation. Trust broken.

No matter what your profession or job, delivering good news is a cherished part of the workday. I loved telling the parents of 18-month-olds, "After shots today, no routine immunizations other than yearly flu shots until the prekindergarten shots at age 4." But I could be making a promise I can't keep. So I'm changing my ways.

Will you?

Much of the anguish around shots is the anticipation of them. So an update…

2013 Immunization Recommendations and Reminders

- The 2013 immunization recommendations have been simplified into one chart for all children from birth to age 18 (used to be 2 charts). It details the timing of shots and necessary intervals between doses for all children. The detailed footnote section explains rationale for all the rules. In my opinion, the 2013 schedule is easier to read and easier to understand.

- **Tetanus, diphtheria, acellular pertussis (Tdap) for every pregnant woman, every pregnancy:** The biggest change to the schedule is the recommendation that all pregnant women get a Tdap shot (protecting against tetanus, diphtheria, and pertussis or whooping cough) in the second half of *each and every pregnancy.* This recommendation was made due to surges in whooping cough infections, epidemics, and a 50-year high in positive cases. Because whooping cough is most risky to newborns, we want pregnant women protected. Ninety percent of those who die from whooping cough are infants. The strategy to vaccinate during every pregnancy takes into account how quickly protection from the vaccine fades after we get it. And the reality is that the vaccine isn't 100% effective. About 80% of those who get it are protected. The best way to protect us all is to have all children and adults up to date on their Tdap.

- New recommendations have been issued for children with immune deficiencies and high-risk conditions (eg, asplenia). See final footnote for details.

- A reminder: boys *and* girls are recommended to have the 3-shot series against HPV starting at age 11. Many parents are very surprised when I tell them this during the visit. (See footnote number 12.)

- Flu shots are recommended for all children aged 6 months to 18 years. Every year your child needs a flu shot or nasal spray, ideally during the late fall.

A few rules for catch-up shots have been updated and simplified. The catch-up schedule is for children behind on immunizations or missing specific shots. Of course, the immunization schedules are updated annually, so be sure to go to http://bit.ly/mdm-VaccineSchedule to see the latest.

FIGURE 1. Recommended immunization schedule for persons aged 0 through 18 years —2013 (for those who fall behind or start late, see the catch-up schedule [Figure 2])

These recommendations must be read with the footnotes that follow. For those who fall behind or start late, provide catch-up vaccination at the earliest opportunity as indicated by the green bars in Figure 1. To determine minimum intervals between doses, see the catch-up schedule (Figure 2). School entry and adolescent vaccine age groups are in bold.

Vaccines	Birth	1 mo	2 mos	4 mos	6 mos	9 mos	12 mos	15 mos	18 mos	19-23 mos	2-3 yrs	**4-6 yrs**	7-10 yrs	**11-12 yrs**	13-15 yrs	16-18 yrs
Hepatitis B¹ (HepB)	1ˢᵗ dose	2ⁿᵈ dose			3ʳᵈ dose											
Rotavirus² (RV) RV-1 (2-dose series); RV-5 (3-dose series)			1ˢᵗ dose	2ⁿᵈ dose	See footnote 2											
Diphtheria, tetanus, & acellular pertussis³ (DTaP: <7 yrs)			1ˢᵗ dose	2ⁿᵈ dose	3ʳᵈ dose			4ᵗʰ dose				5ᵗʰ dose				
Tetanus, diphtheria, & acellular pertussis⁴ (Tdap: ≥7 yrs)														(Tdap)		
Haemophilus influenzae type b⁵ (Hib)			1ˢᵗ dose	2ⁿᵈ dose	See footnote 5		3ʳᵈ or 4ᵗʰ dose see footnote 5									
Pneumococcal conjugate⁶ᵃᶜ (PCV13)			1ˢᵗ dose	2ⁿᵈ dose	3ʳᵈ dose		4ᵗʰ dose									
Pneumococcal polysaccharide⁶ᵇᶜ (PPSV23)																
Inactivated poliovirus⁷ (IPV) (<18years)			1ˢᵗ dose	2ⁿᵈ dose	3ʳᵈ dose							4ᵗʰ dose				
Influenza⁸ (IIV; LAIV) 2 doses for some : see footnote 8					Annual vaccination (IIV only)							Annual vaccination (IIV or LAIV)				
Measles, mumps, rubella⁹ (MMR)							1ˢᵗ dose					2ⁿᵈ dose				
Varicella¹⁰ (VAR)							1ˢᵗ dose					2ⁿᵈ dose				
Hepatitis A¹¹ (HepA)							2 dose series see footnote 11									
Human papillomavirus¹² (HPV2: females only; HPV4: males and females)														(3 dose series)		
Meningococcal¹³ (Hib-MenCY ≥ 6 wks; MCV4-D≥9 mos; MCV4-CRM ≥ 2 yrs.)							see footnote 13							1ˢᵗ dose		booster

Range of recommended ages for all children	Range of recommended ages for catch-up immunization	Range of recommended ages for certain high-risk groups	Range of recommended ages during which catch-up is encouraged and for certain high-risk groups	Not routinely recommended

This schedule includes recommendations in effect as of January 1, 2013. Any dose not administered at the recommended age should be administered at a subsequent visit, when indicated and feasible. The use of a combination vaccine generally is preferred over separate injections of its equivalent component vaccines. Vaccination providers should consult the relevant Advisory Committee on Immunization Practices (ACIP) statement for detailed recommendations, available online at http://www.cdc.gov/vaccines/pubs/acip-list.htm. Clinically significant adverse events that follow vaccination should be reported to the Vaccine Adverse Event Reporting System (VAERS) online (http://www.vaers.hhs.gov) or by telephone (800-822-7967). Suspected cases of vaccine-preventable diseases should be reported to the state or local health department. Additional information, including precautions and contraindications for vaccination, is available from CDC online (http://www.cdc.gov/vaccines) or by telephone (800-CDC-INFO [800-232-4636]).

This schedule is approved by the Advisory Committee on Immunization Practices (http://www.cdc.gov/vaccines/acip/index.html), the American Academy of Pediatrics (http://www.aap.org), the American Academy of Family Physicians (http://www.aafp.org), and the American College of Obstetricians and Gynecologists (http://www.acog.org).

NOTE: The above recommendations must be read along with the footnotes of this schedule.

FIGURE 2. Catch-up immunization schedule for persons aged 4 months through 18 years who start late or who are more than 1 month behind —United States, 2013

The figure below provides catch-up schedules and minimum intervals between doses for children whose vaccinations have been delayed. A vaccine series does not need to be restarted, regardless of the time that has elapsed between doses. Use the section appropriate for the child's age. Always use this table in conjunction with Figure 1 and the footnotes that follow.

Persons aged 4 months through 6 years					
Vaccine	Minimum Age for Dose 1	Minimum Interval Between Doses			
		Dose 1 to dose 2	Dose 2 to dose 3	Dose 3 to dose 4	Dose 4 to dose 5
Hepatitis B[1]	Birth	4 weeks	8 weeks and at least 16 weeks after first dose; minimum age for the final dose is 24 weeks		
Rotavirus[2]	6 weeks	4 weeks	4 weeks[2]		
Diphtheria, tetanus, pertussis[3]	6 weeks	4 weeks	4 weeks	6 months	6 months[3]
Haemophilus influenzae type b[5]	6 weeks	4 weeks if first dose administered at younger than age 12 months 8 weeks (as final dose) if first dose administered at age 12–14 months No further doses needed if first dose administered at age 15 months or older	4 weeks[5] if current age is younger than 12 months 8 weeks (as final dose)[5] If current age is 12 months or older and first dose administered at younger than age 12 months and second dose administered at younger than 15 months No further doses needed if previous dose administered at age 15 months or older	8 weeks (as final dose) This dose only necessary for children aged 12 through 59 months who received 3 doses before age 12 months	
Pneumococcal[8]	6 weeks	4 weeks if first dose administered at younger than age 12 months 8 weeks (as final dose for healthy children) if first dose administered at age 12 months or older or current age 24 through 59 months No further doses needed for healthy children if first dose administered at age 24 months or older	4 weeks if current age is younger than 12 months 8 weeks (as final dose for healthy children) if current age is 12 months or older No further doses needed for healthy children if previous dose administered at age 24 months or older	8 weeks (as final dose) This dose only necessary for children aged 12 through 59 months who received 3 doses before age 12 months or for children at high risk who received 3 doses at any age	
Inactivated poliovirus[7]	6 weeks	4 weeks	4 weeks	6 months[7] minimum age 4 years for final dose	
Meningococcal[13]	6 weeks	8 weeks[13]	see footnote 13	see footnote 13	
Measles, mumps, rubella[9]	12 months	4 weeks			
Varicella[10]	12 months	3 months			
Hepatitis A[11]	12 months	6 months			
Persons aged 7 through 18 years					
Tetanus, diphtheria; tetanus, diphtheria, pertussis[4]	7 years[4]	4 weeks	4 weeks if first dose administered at younger than age 12 months 6 months if first dose administered at 12 months or older	6 months if first dose administered at younger than age 12 months	
Human papillomavirus[12]	9 years	Routine dosing intervals are recommended[12]			
Hepatitis A[11]	12 months	6 months			
Hepatitis B[1]	Birth	4 weeks	8 weeks (and at least 16 weeks after first dose)		
Inactivated poliovirus[7]	6 weeks	4 weeks	4 weeks[7]	6 months[7]	
Meningococcal[13]	6 weeks	8 weeks[13]			
Measles, mumps, rubella[9]	12 months	4 weeks			
Varicella[10]	12 months	3 months if person is younger than age 13 years 4 weeks if person is aged 13 years or older			

NOTE: The above recommendations must be read along with the footnotes of this schedule.

Footnotes — Recommended immunization schedule for persons aged 0 through 18 years—United States, 2013

For further guidance on the use of the vaccines mentioned below, see: http://www.cdc.gov/vaccines/pubs/acip-list.htm.

1. **Hepatitis B (HepB) vaccine. (Minimum age: birth)**
   Routine vaccination:
   At birth
   - Administer monovalent HepB vaccine to all newborns before hospital discharge.
   - For infants born to hepatitis B surface antigen (HBsAg)–positive mothers, administer HepB vaccine and 0.5 mL of hepatitis B immune globulin (HBIG) within 12 hours of birth. These infants should be tested for HBsAg and antibody to HBsAg (anti-HBs) 1 to 2 months after completion of the HepB series, at age 9 through 18 months (preferably at the next well-child visit).
   - If mother's HBsAg status is unknown, within 12 hours of birth administer HepB vaccine to all infants regardless of birth weight. For infants weighing <2,000 grams, administer HBIG in addition to HepB within 12 hours of birth. Determine mother's HBsAg status as soon as possible and, if she is HBsAg-positive, also administer HBIG for infants weighing ≥2,000 grams (no later than age 1 week).
   Doses following the birth dose
   - The second dose should be administered at age 1 or 2 months. Monovalent HepB vaccine should be used for doses administered before age 6 weeks.
   - Infants who did not receive a birth dose should receive 3 doses of a HepB-containing vaccine on a schedule of 0, 1 to 2 months, and 6 months starting as soon as feasible. See Figure 2.
   - The minimum interval between dose 1 and dose 2 is 4 weeks and between dose 2 and 3 is 8 weeks. The final (third or fourth) dose in the HepB vaccine series should be administered no earlier than age 24 weeks, and at least 16 weeks after the first dose.
   - Administration of a total of 4 doses of HepB vaccine is recommended when a combination vaccine containing HepB is administered after the birth dose.
   Catch-up vaccination:
   - Unvaccinated persons should complete a 3-dose series.
   - A 2-dose series (doses separated by at least 4 months) of adult formulation Recombivax HB is licensed for use in children aged 11 through 15 years.
   - For other catch-up issues, see Figure 2.

2. **Rotavirus (RV) vaccines. (Minimum age: 6 weeks for both RV-1 [Rotarix] and RV-5 [RotaTeq]).**
   Routine vaccination:
   - Administer a series of RV vaccine to all infants as follows:
     1. If RV-1 is used, administer a 2-dose series at 2 and 4 months of age.
     2. If RV-5 is used, administer a 3-dose series at ages 2, 4, and 6 months.
     3. If any dose in series was RV-5 or vaccine product is unknown for any dose in the series, a total of 3 doses of RV vaccine should be administered.
   Catch-up vaccination:
   - The maximum age for the first dose in the series is 14 weeks, 6 days.
   - Vaccination should not be initiated for infants aged 15 weeks 0 days or older.
   - The maximum age for the final dose in the series is 8 months, 0 days.
   - If RV-1 (Rotarix) is administered for the first and second doses, a third dose is not indicated.
   - For other catch-up issues, see Figure 2.

3. **Diphtheria and tetanus toxoids and acellular pertussis (DTaP) vaccine. (Minimum age: 6 weeks)**
   Routine vaccination:
   - Administer a 5-dose series of DTaP vaccine at ages 2, 4, 6, 15–18 months, and 4 through 6 years. The fourth dose may be administered as early as age 12 months, provided at least 6 months have elapsed since the third dose.
   Catch-up vaccination:
   - The fifth (booster) dose of DTaP vaccine is not necessary if the fourth dose was administered at age 4 years or older.
   - For other catch-up issues, see Figure 2.

4. **Tetanus and diphtheria toxoids and acellular pertussis (Tdap) vaccine. (Minimum age: 10 years for Boostrix, 11 years for Adacel).**
   Routine vaccination:
   - Administer 1 dose of Tdap vaccine to all adolescents aged 11 through 12 years.
   - Tdap can be administered regardless of the interval since the last tetanus and diphtheria toxoid-containing vaccine.
   - Administer one dose of Tdap vaccine to pregnant adolescents during each pregnancy (preferred during 27 through 36 weeks gestation) regardless of number of years from prior Td or Tdap vaccination.
   Catch-up vaccination:
   - Persons aged 7 through 10 years who are not fully immunized with the childhood DTaP vaccine series, should receive Tdap vaccine as the first dose in the catch-up series; if additional doses are needed, use Td vaccine. For these children, an adolescent Tdap vaccine should not be given.
   - Persons aged 11 through 18 years who have not received Tdap vaccine should receive a dose followed by tetanus and diphtheria toxoids (Td) booster doses every 10 years thereafter.
   - An inadvertent dose of DTaP vaccine administered to children aged 7 through 10 years can count as part of the catch-up series. This dose can count as the adolescent Tdap dose, or the child can later receive a Tdap booster dose at age 11–12 years.
   - For other catch-up issues, see Figure 2.

5. *Haemophilus influenzae* **type b (Hib) conjugate vaccine. (Minimum age: 6 weeks)**
   Routine vaccination:
   - Administer a Hib vaccine primary series and a booster dose to all infants. The primary series doses should be administered at 2, 4, and 6 months of age; however, if PRP-OMP (PedvaxHib or Comvax) is administered at 2 and 4 months of age, a dose at age 6 months is not indicated. One booster dose should be administered at age 12 through15 months.
   - Hiberix (PRP-T) should only be used for the booster (final) dose in children aged 12 months through 4 years, who have received at least 1 dose of Hib.
   Catch-up vaccination:
   - If dose 1 was administered at ages 12-14 months, administer booster (as final dose) at least 8 weeks after dose 1.
   - If the first 2 doses were PRP-OMP (PedvaxHIB or Comvax), and were administered at age 11 months or younger, the third (and final) dose should be administered at age 12 through 15 months and at least 8 weeks after the second dose.
   - If the first dose was administered at age 7 through 11 months, administer the second dose at least 4 weeks later and a final dose at age 12 through 15 months, regardless of Hib vaccine (PRP-T or PRP-OMP) used for first dose.
   - For unvaccinated children aged 15 months or older, administer only 1 dose.
   - For other catch-up issues, see Figure 2.
   Vaccination of persons with high-risk conditions:
   - Hib vaccine is not routinely recommended for patients older than 5 years of age. However one dose of Hib vaccine should be administered to unvaccinated or partially vaccinated persons aged 5 years or older who have leukemia, malignant neoplasms, anatomic or functional asplenia (including sickle cell disease), human immunodeficiency virus (HIV) infection, or other immunocompromising conditions.

6a. **Pneumococcal conjugate vaccine (PCV). (Minimum age: 6 weeks)**
   Routine vaccination:
   - Administer a series of PCV13 vaccine at ages 2, 4, 6 months with a booster at age 12 through 15 months.
   - For children 14 through 59 months who have received an age-appropriate series of 7-valent PCV (PCV7), administer a single supplemental dose of 13-valent PCV (PCV13).
   Catch-up vaccination:
   - Administer 1 dose of PCV13 to all healthy children aged 24 through 59 months who are not completely vaccinated for their age.
   - For other catch-up issues, see Figure 2.
   Vaccination of persons with high-risk conditions:
   - For children aged 24 through 71 months with certain underlying medical conditions (see footnote 6c): administer 1 dose of PCV13 if 3 doses of PCV were received previously, or administer 2 doses of PCV13 at least 8 weeks apart if fewer than 3 doses of PCV were received previously.
   - A single dose of PCV13 may be administered to previously unvaccinated children aged 6 through 18 years who have anatomic or functional asplenia (including sickle cell disease), HIV infection or an immunocompromising condition, cochlear implant or cerebrospinal fluid leak. See MMWR 2010;59 (No. RR-11), available at http://www.cdc.gov/mmwr/pdf/rr/rr5911.pdf.
   - Administer PPSV23 at least 8 weeks after the last dose of PCV to children aged 2 years or older with certain underlying medical conditions (see footnotes 6b and 6c).

6b. **Pneumococcal polysaccharide vaccine (PPSV23). (Minimum age: 2 years)**
   Vaccination of persons with high-risk conditions:
   - Administer PPSV23 at least 8 weeks after the last dose of PCV to children aged 2 years or older with certain underlying medical conditions (see footnote 6c). A single revaccination with PPSV should be administered after 5 years to children with anatomic or functional asplenia (including sickle cell disease) or an immunocompromising condition.

6c. **Medical conditions for which PPSV23 is indicated in children aged 2 years and older and for which use of PCV13 is indicated in children aged 24 through 71 months:**
   - Immunocompetent children with chronic heart disease (particularly cyanotic congenital heart disease and cardiac failure); chronic lung disease (including asthma if treated with high-dose oral corticosteroid therapy), diabetes mellitus; cerebrospinal fluid leaks; or cochlear implant.
   - Children with anatomic or functional asplenia (including sickle cell disease and other hemoglobinopathies, congenital or acquired asplenia, or splenic dysfunction);
   - Children with immunocompromising conditions: HIV infection, chronic renal failure and nephrotic syndrome, diseases associated with treatment with immunosuppressive drugs or radiation therapy, including malignant neoplasms, leukemias, lymphomas and Hodgkin disease; or solid organ transplantation, congenital immunodeficiency.

For further guidance on the use of the vaccines mentioned below, see: http://www.cdc.gov/vaccines/pubs/acip-list.htm.

7. **Inactivated poliovirus vaccine (IPV). (Minimum age: 6 weeks)**
   Routine vaccination:
   - Administer a series of IPV at ages 2, 4, 6–18 months, with a booster at age 4–6 years. The final dose in the series should be administered on or after the fourth birthday and at least 6 months after the previous dose.
   Catch-up vaccination:
   - In the first 6 months of life, minimum age and minimum intervals are only recommended if the person is at risk for imminent exposure to circulating poliovirus (i.e., travel to a polio-endemic region or during an outbreak).
   - If 4 or more doses are administered before age 4 years, an additional dose should be administered at age 4 through 6 years.
   - A fourth dose is not necessary if the third dose was administered at age 4 years or older and at least 6 months after the previous dose.
   - If both OPV and IPV were administered as part of a series, a total of 4 doses should be administered, regardless of the child's current age.
   - IPV is not routinely recommended for U.S. residents aged 18 years or older.
   - For other catch-up issues, see Figure 2.

8. **Influenza vaccines. (Minimum age: 6 months for inactivated influenza vaccine [IIV]; 2 years for live, attenuated influenza vaccine [LAIV])**
   Routine vaccination:
   - Administer influenza vaccine annually to all children beginning at age 6 months. For most healthy, nonpregnant persons aged 2 through 49 years, either LAIV or IIV may be used. However, LAIV should NOT be administered to some persons, including 1) those with asthma, 2) children 2 through 4 years who had wheezing in the past 12 months, or 3) those who have any other underlying medical conditions that predispose them to influenza complications. For all other contraindications to use of LAIV see MMWR 2010; 59 (No. RR-8), available at http://www.cdc.gov/mmwr/pdf/rr/rr5908.pdf.
   - Administer 1 dose to persons aged 9 years and older.
   For children aged 6 months through 8 years:
   - For the 2012–13 season, administer 2 doses (separated by at least 4 weeks) to children who are receiving influenza vaccine for the first time. For additional guidance on dosing guidelines in the 2012 ACIP influenza vaccine recommendations, MMWR 2012; 61: 613–618, available at http://www.cdc.gov/mmwr/pdf/wk/mm6132.pdf.
   - For the 2013–14 season, follow dosing guidelines in the 2013 ACIP influenza vaccine recommendations.

9. **Measles, mumps, and rubella (MMR) vaccine. (Minimum age: 12 months for routine vaccination)**
   Routine vaccination:
   - Administer the first dose of MMR vaccine at age 12 through 15 months, and the second dose at age 4 through 6 years. The second dose may be administered before age 4 years, provided at least 4 weeks have elapsed since the first dose.
   - Administer 1 dose of MMR vaccine to infants aged 6 through 11 months before departure from the United States for international travel. These children should be revaccinated with 2 doses of MMR vaccine, the first at age 12 through 15 months (12 months if the child remains in an area where disease risk is high), and the second dose at least 4 weeks later.
   - Administer 2 doses of MMR vaccine to children aged 12 months and older, before departure from the United States for international travel. The first dose should be administered on or after age 12 months and the second dose at least 4 weeks later.
   Catch-up vaccination:
   - Ensure that all school-aged children and adolescents have had 2 doses of MMR vaccine; the minimum interval between the 2 doses is 4 weeks.

10. **Varicella (VAR) vaccine. (Minimum age: 12 months)**
    Routine vaccination:
    - Administer the first dose of VAR vaccine at age 12 through 15 months, and the second dose at age 4 through 6 years. The second dose may be administered before age 4 years, provided at least 3 months have elapsed since the first dose. If the second dose was administered at least 4 weeks after the first dose, it can be accepted as valid.
    Catch-up vaccination:
    - Ensure that all persons aged 7 through 18 years without evidence of immunity (see MMWR 2007;56 [No. RR-4], available at http://www.cdc.gov/mmwr/pdf/rr/rr5604.pdf) have 2 doses of varicella vaccine. For children aged 7 through 12 years the recommended minimum interval between doses is 3 months (if the second dose was administered at least 4 weeks after the first dose, it can be accepted as valid); for persons aged 13 years and older, the minimum interval between doses is 4 weeks.

11. **Hepatitis A vaccine (HepA). (Minimum age: 12 months)**
    Routine vaccination:

- Initiate the 2-dose HepA vaccine series for children aged 12 through 23 months; separate the 2 doses by 6 to 18 months.
- Children who have received 1 dose of HepA vaccine before age 24 months, should receive a second dose 6 to 18 months after the first dose.
- For any person aged 2 years and older who has not already received the HepA vaccine series, 2 doses of HepA vaccine separated by 6 to 18 months may be administered if immunity against hepatitis A virus infection is desired.
Catch-up vaccination:
- The minimum interval between the two doses is 6 months.
Special populations:
- Administer 2 doses of Hep A vaccine at least 6 months apart to previously unvaccinated persons who live in areas where vaccination programs target older children, or who are at increased risk for infection.

12. **Human papillomavirus (HPV) vaccines. (HPV4 [Gardasil] and HPV2 [Cervarix]). (Minimum age: 9 years)**
    Routine vaccination:
    - Administer a 3-dose series of HPV vaccine on a schedule of 0, 1-2, and 6 months to all adolescents aged 11-12 years. Either HPV4 or HPV2 may be used for females, and only HPV4 may be used for males.
    - The vaccine series can be started beginning at age 9 years.
    - Administer the second dose 1 to 2 months after the first dose and the third dose 6 months after the first dose (at least 24 weeks after the first dose).
    Catch-up vaccination:
    - Administer the vaccine series to females (either HPV2 or HPV4) and males (HPV4) at age 13 through 18 years if not previously vaccinated.
    - Use recommended routine dosing intervals (see above) for vaccine series catch-up.

13. **Meningococcal conjugate vaccines (MCV). (Minimum age: 6 weeks for Hib-MenCY, 9 months for Menactra [MCV4-D], 2 years for Menveo [MCV4-CRM]).**
    Routine vaccination:
    - Administer MCV4 vaccine at age 11–12 years, with a booster dose at age 16 years.
    - Adolescents aged 11 through 18 years with human immunodeficiency virus (HIV) infection should receive a 2-dose primary series of MCV4, with at least 8 weeks between doses. See MMWR 2011; 60:1018–1019 available at: http://www.cdc.gov/mmwr/pdf/wk/mm6030.pdf.
    - For children aged 2 months through 10 years with high-risk conditions, see below.
    Catch-up vaccination:
    - Administer MCV4 vaccine at age 13 through 18 years if not previously vaccinated.
    - If the first dose is administered at age 13 through 15 years, a booster dose should be administered at age 16 through 18 years with a minimum interval of at least 8 weeks between doses.
    - If the first dose is administered at age 16 years or older, a booster dose is not needed.
    - For other catch-up issues, see Figure 2.
    Vaccination of persons with high-risk conditions:
    - For children younger than 19 months of age with anatomic or functional asplenia (including sickle cell disease), administer an infant series of Hib-MenCY at 2, 4, 6, and 12-15 months.
    - For children aged 2 through 18 months with persistent complement component deficiency, administer either an infant series of Hib-MenCY at 2, 4, 6, and 12 through 15 months or a 2-dose primary series of MCV4-D starting at 9 months, with at least 8 weeks between doses. For children aged 19 through 23 months with persistent complement component deficiency who have not received a complete series of Hib-MenCY or MCV4-D, administer 2 primary doses of MCV4-D at least 8 weeks apart.
    - For children aged 24 months and older with persistent complement component deficiency or anatomic or functional asplenia (including sickle cell disease), who have not received a complete series of Hib-MenCY or MCV4-D, administer 2 primary doses of either MCV4-D or MCV4-CRM. If MCV4-D (Menactra) is administered to a child with asplenia (including sickle cell disease), do not administer MCV4-D until 2 years of age and at least 4 weeks after the completion of all PCV13 doses. See MMWR 2011;60:1391–2, available at http://www.cdc.gov/mmwr/pdf/wk/mm6040.pdf.
    - For children aged 9 months and older who are residents of or travelers to countries in the African meningitis belt or to the Hajj, administer an age appropriate formulation and series of MCV4 for protection against serogroups A and W-135. Prior receipt of Hib-MenCY is not sufficient for children traveling to the meningitis belt or the Hajj. See MMWR 2011;60:1391–2, available at http://www.cdc.gov/mmwr/pdf/wk/mm6040.pdf.
    - For children who are present during outbreaks caused by a vaccine serogroup, administer or complete an age and formulation-appropriate series of Hib-MenCY or MCV4.
    - For booster doses among persons with high-risk conditions refer to http://www.cdc.gov/vaccines/pubs/acip-list.htm#mening.

Additional information
- For contraindications and precautions to use of a vaccine and for additional information regarding that vaccine, vaccination providers should consult the relevant ACIP statement available online at http://www.cdc.gov/vaccines/pubs/acip-list.htm.
- For the purposes of calculating intervals between doses, 4 weeks = 28 days. Intervals of 4 months or greater are determined by calendar date.
- Information on travel vaccine requirements and recommendations is available at http://wwwnc.cdc.gov/travel/page/vaccinations.htm.
- For vaccination of persons with primary and secondary immunodeficiencies, see Table 13, "Vaccination of persons with primary and secondary immunodeficiencies," in General Recommendations on Immunization (ACIP), available at http://www.cdc.gov/mmwr/preview/mmwrhtml/rr6002a1.htm; and American Academy of Pediatrics. Immunization in Special Clinical Circumstances. In: Pickering LK, Baker CJ, Kimberlin DW, Long SS eds. Red book: 2012 report of the Committee on Infectious Diseases. 29th ed. Elk Grove Village, IL: American Academy of Pediatrics.

Human Papillomavirus

In 2006, I entered pediatric practice. It was the same year that the Advisory Committee on Immunization Practices recommended to start giving 11-year-old girls the human papillomavirus (HPV) vaccine. Therefore, I've really never practiced pediatrics (outside of my training) without the ability to offer up immunization and protection against HPV; I've been discussing this for about 7 years. We now give HPV shots to boys and girls because it's so common—about 50% of all adults who are sexually active will get one form of HPV in their lifetime.

Human papillomavirus can come into our bodies and do no harm. But it also can come into our bodies and cause vaginal, penis, anal, and oral/throat warts. Other strains of HPV cause changes in the cervix that can lead to cervical cancer and can rarely lead to penile and/or tongue/throat cancer. Teens and adults can get HPV from oral, vaginal, or anal sex. *Condoms don't provide 100% protection from getting it.*

Great News: Being protected (by the HPV shot) doesn't trigger risky sexual behaviors in teens.

Nice to have an immunization to protect against the potential development of such disfiguring, embarrassing, and uncomfortable lesions. And what a windfall to have a vaccine that prevents cancer. I often say to my patients, "If my grandmother only knew that I'd see the day where we could prevent cancer." I mean it—if she only could have seen the day (she died in the late 1980s).

The reality is that parents of teenaged girls have consistently been hesitant about getting the HPV vaccine in my office. Over the last 6 years, hesitancy around getting HPV vaccine has lessened, but many of my patients' parents have told me that they don't want their girls or boys to feel that getting the shots is a green light for sexual activity. And many have worried that having their girls immunized will make them more likely to engage in earlier sexual activity.

Parents often say, "But she's only 11!" or "We know she isn't going to have sex before marriage," or "He's just so young." Reality is, the best way to protect girls and boys from HPV is to have them develop immunity (responding to the HPV 3-shot series takes 6 months) *before* ever having any sexual contact. Even if they are just starting to develop breasts or their penis is just starting to grow, age 11 can be a great time to start the HPV series so that teens have completed and responded to all 3 shots by the time they are sexually active. There is no reason to wait to get HPV shots. The risks are no lower for a 15-year-old when compared with an 11-year-old.

Only 13% of 15-year-olds have had sex. But 70% of 19-year-olds have. We want all teens protected against HPV prior to any sexual contact.

A study in the November 2012 *Pediatrics* proves that the concern about early sexual activity after the HPV shot is not the reality. It's not only fantastic news, it's exceedingly reassuring for the concerns many parents have.

HPV Vaccination Does Not Change Sexual Behavior

At the 11-year visit, we now offer 3 shots to girls and boys: HPV; tetanus, diphtheria, acellular pertussis (Tdap); and meningococcal conjugate (MCV4). The HPV vaccine has 2 follow-up booster doses: one shot 2 months later and one shot 6 months after the first.

Researchers studied nearly 500 11- to 12-year-old girls who had received HPV vaccine (at least one dose). They compared those girls with 900 other girls who only received Tdap and MCV4 at their 11-year well-child appointment. All 1,400 girls were followed for 3 years. Researchers then compared testing, diagnosis, and counseling outcomes when it came to sexual activity, sexually transmitted infections (STIs), and pregnancy (visits to the doctor for any pregnancy or STI testing or diagnosis or visits for birth control counseling).

Girls who received HPV shots were no different than girls who didn't.

Researchers concluded that HPV vaccine was not related to any "sexual-activity outcome" rates. Meaning, getting the HPV shot didn't endorse sexual activity and thus didn't lead to more STIs, unintended pregnancies, or coming into the office for birth control.

Tips for Teens Getting Their 11-Year Shots

- Bring a cell phone, smartphone, tablet, or enticing magazine along with you to the clinic.
- The HPV vaccine really stings when it goes in. Most all teens report this back to me! This is in part because of the high salt concentration in the solution in the injection. Although telling your teen, "This shot is really going to hurt," won't help and will likely only increase anxiety, providing support for and acknowledgment of the discomfort during and after the shot is very helpful. Also, help distract your teen during the shot (use a smartphone, tell a story or joke, ask your teen about prom—something!). And if your teen is anxious or nervous, have your teen wait 10 to 15 minutes after getting the shot to prevent your teen from getting woozy or fainting. Teens often feel woozy or even faint after any shot during the teen years.
- Many parents are concerned about shots for STIs. Do your best to ask your teen's doctor or nurse about fears or worries you have. You're certainly not alone in being queasy about your teen potentially having sex someday.
- **Fear of needles?** If you teen has a fear of needles, don't hesitate to talk to your child's clinician about the fear and get him or her on board to help. Teens are often extremely anxious but nervous to admit it.
- **Finish the series:** Make that first poke worth it! The best way to protect your teen (or yourself) from getting HPV is to finish all 3 shots in the series. Don't forget to return to the nurse or medical assistant for the 2-month and 6-month boosters! Many girls and boys start the series and don't finish, thus leaving them exposed and vulnerable to HPV when they are sexually active. Teens have a bad track record for all their shots but the worst record when it comes to finishing HPV shots.

Mama Doc Vitals

Fact: The Centers for Disease Control and Prevention (CDC) reports that human papillomavirus (HPV) immunization rates are lower for younger girls (age 11 and 12 years) than older teens—many girls aren't getting their shots when recommended. Getting the shot early will protect girls from ever getting the virus.

Human papillomavirus causes cervical cancer, penile and anal cancers, and oral and throat cancers. It also causes warts in the genital and anal area.

Timeline Trouble: In 2006, we started to give quadrivalent (4 strains) vaccine to girls to prevent 70% of cervical cancers caused by HPV. Then in 2010, full license from the US Food and Drug Administration was granted in the United States to immunize and protect boys from anal cancer. This may lead the public to doubt that boys need it.

Human papillomavirus causes warts and cervical cancer. But 8,000 boys and men in the United States develop cancers annually caused by HPV. Six thousand of these male cancers are oral and throat lesions.

Girls will still need Papanicolaou tests ("Pap smears") throughout adulthood after having HPV vaccine because some cervical cancers (20%–30%) develop from causes other than HPV.

Link: Here are data from the CDC: http://bit.ly/mdm-TeenVaccines.

Part 4

Work-Life Balance/Mothering

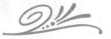

KEEPING THE BALANCE

An increasing number of women are now the primary or sole breadwinners of their household—and yet mothers feel pressure to "do it all," hearing conflicting information in the media, at work, and at home. Here's a look at the current challenges and joys of balancing the job of raising a child while also working outside the home.

THE STATE OF THE WORKING MOM

40%
of women are now the primary or sole breadwinners in the US.

61%
of mothers work at home.

2011 Median Family Incomes

$80,000
Wife is primary breadwinner.

$78,000
Husband is primary breadwinner.

$70,000
Spouses' incomes are about the same.

HOW HAPPY ARE WORKING MOMS COMPARED WITH STAY-AT-HOME MOMS?

85%
Working mothers who say they are "very happy" or "pretty happy"

80%
Stay-at-home mothers who say they are "very happy" or "pretty happy"

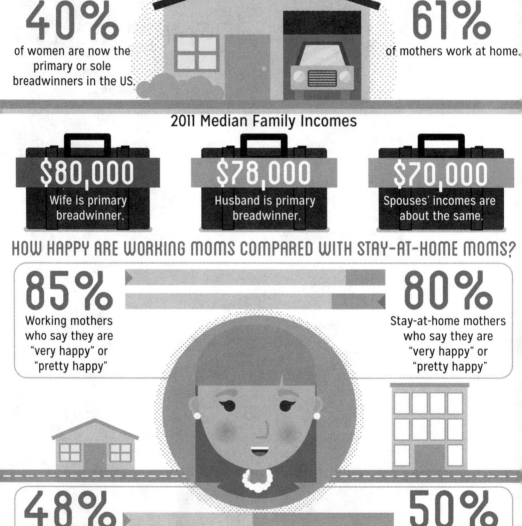

48%
Working mothers who say they feel stressed

50%
Stay-at-home mothers who say they feel stressed

WE'RE MORE SIMILAR THAN WE THOUGHT!

WE CAN DO BETTER.

While the number of working mothers grows,
significant inequities remain that we must work to fix.

Inequality Among Working Mothers

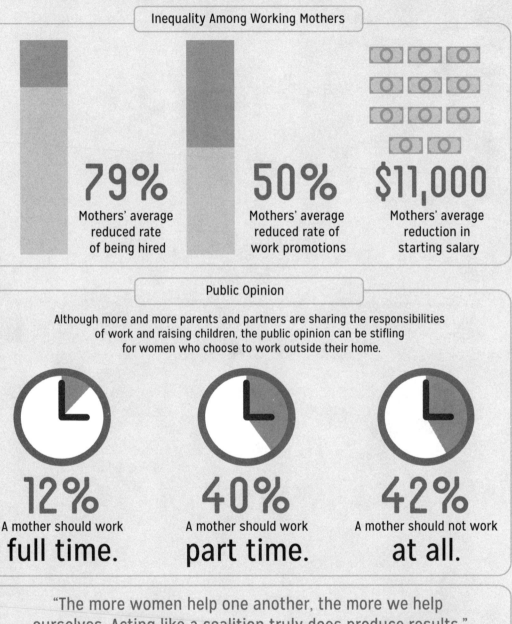

79%
Mothers' average
reduced rate
of being hired

50%
Mothers' average
reduced rate of
work promotions

$11,000
Mothers' average
reduction in
starting salary

Public Opinion

Although more and more parents and partners are sharing the responsibilities
of work and raising children, the public opinion can be stifling
for women who choose to work outside their home.

12%
A mother should work
full time.

40%
A mother should work
part time.

42%
A mother should not work
at all.

"The more women help one another, the more we help
ourselves. Acting like a coalition truly does produce results."
- Sheryl Sandberg
Lean In: Women, Work, and the Will to Lead

Sources
* www.gallup.com/poll/154685/Stay-Home-Moms-Report-Depression-Sadness-Anger.aspx *
* www.statisticbrain.com/working-mother-statistics *
* www.pewsocialtrends.org/2013/05/29/breadwinner-moms *

Part 4
Work-Life Balance/Mothering

Introduction

There's something enormously fallible about being a parent. Moments when we mess up and fess up to our regrets; moments of bad decisions and acknowledgment of our naive inexperience. See, each and every day we're asked to parent a child who's a little older, and we start a job we've never done before. We're always novices, a little bit.

I've had some low moments at the edge of the pool. When I describe them, you may not think they are such a big deal. You'll perhaps tilt your head and wonder why it's been so hard for me. I realized finally that it's because I keep letting myself down, keep attempting to do the right thing but can't seem to align myself with the right strategy. I keep failing and flailing in trying to wrestle with my 5-year-old's demands and resistance. And I keep failing at reaching the goal I once desired.

He's entirely different than my 7-year-old. And that's the rub. Nothing I learned 2 years prior to my 5-year-old's birth helps me get him in the swimming pool when he refuses.

For some reason, perhaps anxiety, he's started to refuse all the activities he is signed up to do—ballet, swimming lessons, soccer. He refuses even though he has expressed and displayed enormous joy while at these activities and asked us to sign him up. And there's something about his insistence simultaneous with his resistance and the power with which he stands behind his ideas that fills me with rage.

Rage.

It's rage I feel sometimes when I haul out of work, race home, get him ready for the activity, and then we find ourselves standing on the edge of the pool with one little boy refusing to jump. Metaphors aside, the precipice and conflict at the moment our toes are at the edge of the deep end make me furious.

And it's not just about the activity.

And it's not just the reality that he has said he loves to swim.

And it's not just about the money we paid for the lessons.

And it's not just about the time I take off from work to get him to the pool on time.

And it's not just that I love watching him enjoy his class and confidence in water.

The true source of my rage lies a little in between all those things. In the space where he has his hook right in me—that space and niche of getting my goat. Defying what's expected.

As I detail in "Mindful Parenting" (Chapter 37, page 157), I loved being reminded by Jon Kabat-Zinn, PhD, in a talk I attended on mindfulness that those we love the most also inspire the most ire. Oh, I love my Oden desperately, yet hate the conflicts that only a 5-year-old dreams up on the pool deck.

One pediatrician and friend warned me once about the mounting smarts and complex tantrums during the early school years, saying, "Yeah—there's the terrible twos, the trying threes, and the f-ing fours and fives!"

The pool and swimming-lesson territory has history for me. A comment passed on by another mother about 3 years ago lingers and sets the stage for the rage and the complex balance I'm always striving for. I want to be entirely present, witness the awe-inspiring fortune of raising a child, but also work as a doctor and contribute to my community. I want to be a stay-at-home mom and a pediatrician. It's perhaps cloning that would be most ideal. All these conversations about having it all really do make me stumble.

See, the pool is not my favorite place. Some years ago I scrambled into the dressing room at the pool with the boys. A colleague's wife (and friend) and her 2 children were already there. When she saw me and the boys, she said, "Wendy Sue, you must not know what to do with yourself being so early today."

Do you get it? Do you get that I'd raced home from clinic, scooped up the boys, changed them into swimsuits, frantically parked the car, trying to "do it all" on time? That the one and only time I succeed in exceeding the clock, I get reprimanded and teased by a mom who wasn't in a rush? And is always on time. Boy, it stung.

And that's what this part of the book explores. The jungle of the stay-at-home mom/working mom dialogue and the natural observations in my head as a pediatrician. How the balance for me and so many working parents is elusive and ever-changing as we mature as parents and as our children's needs and development shift.

My favorite chapter is the last (*"Time* Magazine and the Mommy Middle Road," page 369).

72

Competitive Parenting

Raising children in a world full of accessible opinions is a funny thing. Everyone seems to have an idea about how to do this right. Stay home, work full time, work part time, return to work, cry to sleep, not cry to sleep, pacifier, no pacifier…the recipe for each of us is different, of course. Often we're all right in what we're doing, from picking out baby food to enrolling our child in preschool. But it doesn't always feel that way when a barrage of comments and advice from relatives, friends, and people in the supermarket hits us in the shins. What people say about how we care for our children hurts far more than salt in a wound. Editorials on our parenting can seriously linger.

I started calling this *competitive parenthood* after I talked with Liz Szabo at *USA Today* about this challenge. She wrote a popular article called, "Why do mothers judge one another and their parenting?" in which she quoted me and a number of other moms and doctors about our experiences.

Most people who read the article even now tell me that it makes them feel better.

I got halfway through the book *Instinctive Parenting: Trusting Ourselves to Raise Good Kids* by Ada Calhoun. The introduction and first few chapters were mesmerizing. I found myself nodding, laughing, and gasping out loud— it seemed she and I were so aligned. She made me feel like we really all can do this perfectly. Armed with instincts, we really can help our children thrive. But then about 10 chapters in, it started to feel like even in a book about trusting yourself, not the voices in the news/baby books/neighborhood/playground, she had a story to tell and one that was instructive. Not steeped in judgment, but instructive. As if in parenting, to steel ourselves into trusting our own instincts, we may have to believe in the demonization of the other side or opinion. Maybe it's simply instinctual to feel righteous about how you do it. Maybe it inspires the confidence we all need?

Here's how I see it.

- Competitive parenting abounds. We all know what it feels like to be judged or evaluated in what we do. Yet we become righteous toward others when we're successful in a task/method and feel everyone else should do the same.

This makes sense and is how we "get through." But often there is far more than one "right" way to do things.

- As a pediatrician I see parents for checkups every day I'm in clinic. *Every parent has some concern about how to care for, protect, and raise his or her child.* Don't let other parents fool you; we all have questions about how to do this well.

- Besides a few important safety measures (eg, back to sleep for infant sleep, using car seats properly, getting lifesaving vaccines, securing the furniture to the walls), most parenting issues have multiple right answers. That is, there are many ways to all of this that are "right." I agree with Ada—trusting your own instincts, not the instincts of others, is the best way to proceed. But as I'll share, in my opinion there are a few ways our instincts serve us poorly.

- Listening to friends and family who are raising children may be far more important than telling. Employing a virtual muzzle to stifle opinions might help all of us! As my mother-in-law wisely says, "If someone isn't asking for advice, whatever advice you provide will be perceived as criticism."

- Often when we become judgmental of other parents, it's because we're evaluating our own choices.

- A big debate and source of sour feelings come around the decision to stay home versus work while raising families. This decision and tension are usually more challenging for women. From the time you return to work (or don't) from maternity leave, there will be people telling you how to do it right. The national dialogue about "having it all" pulses again and again.

- Only you will know the perfect balance of work and time at home for yourself. Your recipe for balance will likely not be the same as even those you respect or emulate. Often you won't know what is perfect right away. Have patience with your decisions; you can always change your mind. The "perfect" balance may remain elusive and feel like a moving target as your children grow and change. That part is normal too.

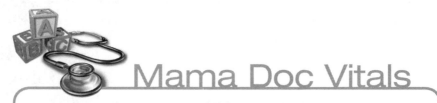

Mama Doc Vitals

Link: The *USA Today* article: http://bit.ly/mdm-MommyWars

The Working Mom Wonders, "What Am I Doing?"

I get caught in a recurring cloud of indecision and doubt. As I raise my boys and as they change what they seek and what they need, I find myself spinning around to grab the cup of milk or the steering wheel, muttering, "What am I doing?"

When the boys were 20 months and 3 years of age, I distinctly got caught in the cycle of doubt. Although the specifics are different each and every year, the cycle of wondering what I am doing with my work and what I'm doing with my family bubbles up.

I constantly look at other parents and learn from their choices.

I do fall back perseverating on how to do this right. Life, I mean. How to work, how to parent, and how to, at some point, care for myself amid the demands.

The issue of balance between work and parenting while trying to contribute to the world and use my skills seems germane for most of my friends too. I never quite know what will trip me up, triggering a reevaluation. But it comes up. Quarterly, let's say, like state taxes.

There are days I am astonished by my opportunities and the children I get to take care of. And days when I am so delighted by my own children, I still cry when I leave for work sometimes. And then there are days I question if I have the stamina to endure. There are days that by the end of clinic, I'm so tired my eyes appear bloodshot. My medical assistant has more than once taken my temperature, suggesting I was likely ill. It's usually normal. But, point is, it happens; I get really tired just like every other working parent.

The real trouble is this: I like my days in clinic and the things I discover. Recently I was able to diagnose a broken bone previously missed in a 2-week-old, support a teenager with a new diagnosis of depression, and complete 20+ well-child checkups. I love it. But tired and missing my boys, yes. See, this would be far easier if I was only pulled in one direction. It's just not how it works for me; I have tugs on each limb.

The endless tug-of-war between arguments for those who stay at home and those who work while raising kids goes on and on in my head. Specifically, though, the retreat back to this issue of balance between work and home—and my current decision to work (a lot)–was spawned by 4 things.

- A blog post I read, now 2 months ago, has lingered. The post really was about how we all come to our own decisions. Yet the message on Twitter that led me to the article said, "Family comes first for some who have finished residency." The blog post details how some doctors choose to stay home with their children, even after completing rigorous medical training. The post wasn't written by the obstetrician who decided to stay home with her children; rather, it was written by a working colleague. Funny, I thought. And when I read it the first time I was headed out the door for one of my long clinic days where I work well past 8:00 pm. The blog post ruined my day. Maybe it was the title of the post that ruined my day. Just because I work doesn't mean my family doesn't come first! My rebuttal, now years later, would be entitled, "Family comes first for some who have finished residency," except it would describe what I do too. See, my family does come first even when I'm at work. When we're off helping others, it's devastating when people challenge our love and dedication to our own.
- Another conversation with a physician friend (who at the time was a self-declared stay-at-home mom) also set me back. After a whole conversation in which my work *didn't* come up as we chatted about our kids, she asked, "Are you and Jonathan OK?" The tone of the question seemed to imply pity for our circumstance of working while raising our boys. I was taken aback. See, we were, we are, we will be OK. We exceed OK. We're ecstatic about our lives and opportunities at work. The question, gowned in judgment, made my heart hurt and made me question, yet again, was I doing this all right? Although pity is unlikely what she implied, it's how I took it and how I remember it. And doubt lingers.
- While the boys have been young, I've been lucky enough to work from home writing a few days a week. At 20 months, O's language was launching, rocket style. In tough moments (you know, like wanting a toy), he's been instantly calling out, "Mommy!" It takes a lot in me not to go running. And hearing this from upstairs had me wondering.
- The judgment from grandmas and moms farther down the parenting road can silence us. When once we saw an old family friend, she asked about work—my practice, writing and blogging, etc. I told her how much I was working, quantifying it in hours—about 60 to 70 hours a week. Her

response: "Does that leave you any time to parent?" Of course it does, I protested. It just doesn't leave me time to sleep. The comment, steeped in judgment, pierced me. And of course, it lingers too.

Fortunately, wisdom from parents and refreshing new perspectives save us all.

WendySueSwanson MD @SeattleMamaDoc
The complexity of #worklifebalance is that imbalance sometimes highlights meaning.

For one of Oden's well-child checkups, I took the morning off (minus a 7:00 am interview) and spent it with the boys. I did mom-type things—a trip to Finn's school, a stop at the park, got the car washed, and went to the grocery store. Although there is nothing romantic about the list, the change in pace and in the day was a delightful shift for me. Then Oden and I sailed into the pediatric clinic for his checkup.

Oden's pediatrician did his checkup. Then she asked how I was. I launched into the aforementioned topic about my struggle about balance. I was describing how many people over the last 6 months have *warned me*. They say things like, "Your boys will only be young once," or, "Your boys want you around now but won't want you around later." I explained to her how it has me all caught up and spiderwebbed. That the comments and quandary have been angst-inducing and guilt-inspiring. And how I am always chewing on the fact that no one says this to my husband.

But then, just as I was tearing up and reentering the cloud, a sunbeam shot through. O's pediatrician (a mom of 3) said, "Oh no, that's not true. Your boys will always want you around, when they are teenagers and grown-ups too." She went on to explain her specifics and rationale. Her experience, her success, and her own regrets.

All of a sudden the cloud was gone. I was affirmed and understood again and so appreciative that she made the decision to go to work too.

74

Only One Decision

When becoming a parent, we make a big choice. One enormous decision. Hello, understatement of the century. I remember my father-in-law saying, "There's a freight train coming," just before Finn was born. Yes, thunderous and steamy, I was ushered into a new world in December 2006, when my first freight train hit. And although I now may be billowing steam and coal, motherhood is the most astounding segment of my life thus far.

I read a blog post written by an obstetrician, Amy Tuteur, MD, who authors the blog, "The Skeptical OB." We may hum on the same wavelength. She says that "…good mothering is about choosing motherhood and not about mothering choices."

When I read her post, I nearly held my breath. Then I reread it again a few times. So much of what she says makes sense to me and hits on my recurring theme about parenting in the world of opinion—the reality that there is no manual, no right or correct way to parent. There is no needed judgment and guilt about our choices. Love and commitment to our children may be the only prerequisites for success. I found Dr Tuteur's blog post about choosing parenting on a popular medical blog this past weekend.

I felt like she was channeling my thoughts.

At one point she says, "My fundamental objection to the philosophies of natural childbirth and attachment parenting is not the emphasis that they place on mothering; I object to the fact that they privilege specific mothering choices over others."

Hallelujah. Read her entire post on the next page.

Choosing mothering vs. mothering choices

Since the subtext of the natural childbirth and attachment parenting movements is the notion of the good mother, it's worth asking what makes a good mother. My whole approach to writing about childbirth and mothering choices is based my rejection of currently popular beliefs about good mothering. Simply put, I believe that good mothering is about choosing mothering and not about mothering choices.

What does choosing mothering mean? It means actively embracing the role of caretaker, confidante, educator and moral guide that mothering entails. It means worrying, planning, consulting, advising and ultimately letting go. Should he be the youngest in kindergarten or wait a year and be the oldest? How should she handle the playground teasing? Am I expecting too much from him or does he have a learning disability? Should I let her go to the dance with the older boy or is she still too vulnerable?

It is kissing the boo-boos, helping them face the fears, stepping aside and allowing them to talk to the doctor in private when they are old enough. It is piano lessons, orthodontia, religious services, holiday celebrations. It is not responding when she says "I hate you" and never failing to respond when you see him teasing another child. It is hard, damn hard, with weeks or months that leave you exhausted or emotionally drained. Yet it is also rewarding at the deepest level, forging a bond to last a lifetime, launching a happy young adult into the world.

It is NOT about specific mothering choices. Breast or bottle? That's the mother's choice and nobody else's business. Natural childbirth? Irrelevant. Baby wearing? It depends on the baby and on the mother. Extended breastfeeding? Meaningless in the long run (and often in the short run, too).

How do we know a woman is a good mother? We know because she cares; she cares about her children and cares about the impact that she is having on those children. To love a child is to choose mothering. In contrast, specific mothering choices have nothing to do with love, because there is not only one way to express love.

My fundamental objection to the philosophies of natural childbirth and attachment parenting is not the emphasis that they place on mothering; I object to the fact that they privilege specific mothering choices over others. In other words, adherents believe their own mothering choices proclaim their "goodness" and that different choices on the part of other mothers identify them as bad mothers.

Instead of viewing mothering as a service they willingly give their children, they view it as a social identity that they construct for themselves, boosting their own egos in the process. That's why discussions about NCB, breastfeeding and attachment parenting are such a source of discord between women. None of those discussions are about the best way to mother a baby; they're all about who is the best mother. It may seem like a trivial difference, but it is an immense difference and most women recognize it as such.

The most critical ingredient of good mothering is love. A child who is loved has the advantage over any other child, regardless of the specific parenting choices his mother made. It's time to acknowledge and value the power of choosing motherhood and stop judging other women based on mothering choices.

~ Amy Tuteur, MD. Reprinted with permission.

75

Doctor, Daughter, Mother, and Wife: 4 Corners

I wrote this the day before my mom started chemotherapy. I realized something.

It feels like my 2 feet are reaching to stand in 4 separate corners. Doctor, Daughter, Mom, and Wife. Four corners. Except nothing about the sky looks like Utah right now.

I'm caught in the middle of a generational sandwich. I've started to understand that taking care of those older than me and those younger than me (while, at the same time, attempting to tend to myself) may define adulthood. This week I awoke to the sobering reality that I'm a real grown-up. Good morning, Sunday; meet me, Grown-up number 221005. It seems I've finally earned the title.

Titles tend to follow set milestones in life. You finish your 12th year and you're a teenager. Eighteen and you're a voter. Finish college, you're an adult. Finish medical school and they call you doctor. Yet often, these titles are granted asynchronously from earnest accomplishment or achievements.

Take the example of being called "Doctor." When I was a resident working in the neonatal intensive care unit (NICU), one supervising physician set me straight. After an absolutely wretched night that I will remember for the rest of my life, we sat down to review charts at about 8:00 am. I'd been up all night as a senior resident caring for premature infants, running to resuscitate premature babies at deliveries, assisting and working with nurses in the NICU, and witnessing the death of 2 infants. It was a tragic night. I'd just filled out a death certificate and tidied up my to-do list for the morning when we sat down to review our patients. My sage attending said, "Dr Swanson, every single day, someone calls you 'Doctor.' Every once in a while, you earn the title."

It turns out that this might be another opportunity for me to earn my other title, Daughter.

Up to this point, I've been fairly academic, intellectual, and "doctorly" about my mom's cancer diagnosis. I hide out in the numbers and the science of her disease. Sometimes it's an easier place to be.

The day she started chemotherapy, I had to venture out of the decimal points with my mom as daughter. At the cancer center, like my mom, I will always hope and pray for the best while I wait for little miracles. But I am also scared. So, Doctor is in there, but Daughter and Grown-up sit more squarely in the center.

I can do this, Mom. Without hesitation. So can you.

Ever since I finished med school, my mom has had my name labeled in her e-mail, "Wendy Sue, MD, MBE, MDDtD." MDDtD: My Darling Daughter the Doctor. Thanks for the confidence in my dual roles, Mom; I hope never to let you down.

She-Woman Wednesday

Our nanny called in sick one day when the boys were really young. I remember that surviving the chaos fueled me with energy. I felt like a She-Woman (think gender equal of He-Man circa 1988) after making it through the day. Maybe it's more She-Ra. Between the hours of 7:50 am when I got the call and 5:50 pm when I sat down to dinner with my little boys, I

- Kissed the husband good-bye.
- Convinced Grandma to watch Oden for the day.
- Packed up Oden's things, along with the dog, and threw them (OK, not really) in the car.
- Got Finn ready.
- Dropped Luna (the dog) and Oden (the boy) off at Grandma's house.
- Took Finn to day number 2 of preschool. He clung, cried, clawed for me to stay. Heartbreaking.
- Arrived at Children's Hospital by 9:00 am. Thank you very much. I take a bow.
- Finally published a blog post on chlorine, drowning, swimming lessons, and my opinions on a bad study.
- Returned e-mails. Many.
- Realized I forgot my iPhone at home. Then realized I sat at a desk that had no phone.
- Realized I was nearly undetectable for a few hours. Motivating. Got work done.
- Called Grandma to make sure Oden was OK; informed her I had no phone and didn't have my pager on. She was going to have to fend for herself.
- Went to a local radio station downtown and recorded public service announcements. This only after my genius decision to have milk for lunch for the first time in 2 decades. Cleared my throat an extra 12 times while recording.
- Returned more e-mails; went to meetings.
- Corrected spelling mistakes. Note: spell-check has officially ruined the spelling space that once, very long ago, existed in my brain.

- Picked up Finn. Hurrah!
- Picked up Oden at Grandma's. Double hurrah!
- Picked up Luna (the dog). Woof.
- Arrived home and made dinner for the boys. Annie's Mac & Cheese, broccolini, ham, palm hearts, apple, and avocado. Yes, this felt gourmet under the circumstances.

And yes, I am patting myself on the back.

I do feel as though it would have been easier to lift up the left corner of our house for 3 minutes.

You know you have your He-Man/She-Woman/She-Ra–equivalent moments too. When no one else knows what a Herculean task it was just to get your body to work. Some morning disaster like kid vomit, or the car breaking down, or the car not starting, or no milk in house, or no child care, or kid spits up on the first 2 outfits you put on, or power out, or ice storm and the car door is sealed shut, or phone call with bad news, or, ummm, I dunno, the dog ran off. But you find your Master of the Universe from within and you triumph, arriving at work on time. Or at a reasonable time. You slip in, grab your pencil, and put your head down as if it were nothing. As if you'd had a long shower and a nice breakfast, read the paper, sipped a cappuccino, and strolled into work while chatting on the phone. Yup. You got 'em fooled.

Hopefully I did too.

WendySueSwanson MD @SeattleMamaDoc

"Superwoman is the adversary of the woman's movement."
–Gloria Steinem via @sherylsandberg in Lean In #worklifebalance

77

Every Illness, a Love Story

One magical thing I see while working in health care is the love story. Each and every child who encounters a diagnosis or illness spawns a collection of love stories around them. The stories come spontaneously from parents, siblings, friends, nurses, doctors, community, and peers. It all happens organically and sometimes it happens without notice. Babies cling to their parents when they ache; parents cling to their children when they worry. And the acknowledgment of mortality can stun us into living in the present moment—a miraculous gift. With the onset of an illness or injury, a series of love stories begins in earnest around every child as we all seem to fall in love again.

It may be innate; I think it's impossible to stop these love stories from unfolding when a child is ill.

A physician colleague once pointed out to me that only 2 things bring you to the doctor: 1) anxiety about an illness (or wanting to prevent one) and 2) pain. With children, when either (anxiety or pain) are present, a love story erupts around them. Immediately and passionately, those who care for children and witness their lives will work tirelessly to ease pain and suffering. In it, their love unfolds.

I've just realized that a love story is always a part of the history of present illness. Here's why.

Recently a friend shared with me a new, life-threatening diagnosis his child had received. He invited me into a Facebook group designed for his family to track their journey and chronicle their experiences, support their son, and coordinate their efforts. The Facebook group is primarily authored and updated by the boy's mother. For 100+ days I read a near-daily update on their boy's medical condition, their month-plus stay in the hospital, and their family experience of their son's illness—the days of isolation in the hospital, the homecomings, the readmissions, the remarkable intimacy between a parent and child, the weighted worry, and the hope that comes with each brilliant step toward a cure. But more than anything, stronger than any medical detail documented, this family journals its love. I've come to see the Facebook group as a beautiful love story. A mother's and father's love, a love for their son's present and his future, a love for God, a love for community, a love for family, and a love for the return of routine.

Witnessing this incredible family embrace their son and love one another is changing the way I think about doctoring and my own life as a parent. I'm exceptionally fortunate to read their love story and have the opportunity to think and pray for them every single day.

Every illness, a love story.

It is in this way that I believe social tools and networks are transforming our experience of illness, parenting, doctoring, caregiving, loving, and living our lives. Like my patients' stories, this love story has changed mine. And it is these challenges and illnesses that indeed provide us wisdom while ultimately making us much stronger.

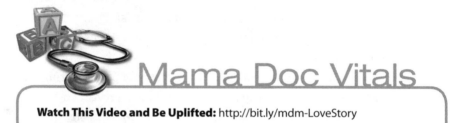

Mama Doc Vitals

Watch This Video and Be Uplifted: http://bit.ly/mdm-LoveStory

78

The Juggle: Working and Breastfeeding

A study in *Pediatrics* highlighting the importance of breastfeeding and the challenges for working moms was published in 2009. It circulated through a business journal and got some more attention.

I read the study. Then I reread it a number of times. I talk about breastfeeding with moms and parents in clinic every day I'm in the office. I certainly know the challenges of trying to breastfeed through a transition back to work. I also know how hard it is not to be able to do what you set out to do.

I had my go. With my first son, I saw about 9 lactation consultants in the first week. I am not exaggerating. Me with those women hovering over me trying to help while my little man screamed his head off. It was the beginning of motherhood for me. It was tense and I was a bit frantic.

I breastfed, finger-fed, pumped breast milk, finger-fed, breastfed, then pumped my way into a sleepless oblivion. One month into this circus, I was hospitalized for 4 days with a severe breast infection that required intravenous antibiotics. This didn't stop me. I had set out to breastfeed after learning the health benefits, waiting for my baby, and supporting numerous moms to do the same. I ended up exclusively pumping breast milk until my son was almost 5 months old. By then, my supply was nearly gone, my time with the pump had me spinning, and I had no place at work I felt comfortable pumping. I'd been offered one of the patient examination rooms (with no lock on the door) to pump and I didn't stand up for something more ideal...I was new there. I threw in the towel. Teary eyed and filled with failure, I gave in to being with my son over the pump and started to feed him formula.

I didn't make it to 12 months like I had wanted. I would have been pleased with even 6. But I didn't make it. I did learn a lot along the way, though. And it's certainly clear to me now that I needed to find more of the right people to help support me at home and in my work space.

Here's my take when it comes to breastfeeding and working. There is math involved.

I think working moms who are able to breastfeed and maintain their milk supply have a fairly onerous task. It's entirely doable. Stating this reality doesn't mean I don't support or believe that breast milk is optimal. But I think it's exhausting to go back to work with a newborn. It can be delightful and exhausting to breastfeed a newborn. The combination and juggling of both roles can be intimidating as a working mom. In my opinion, moms who are trying to breastfeed really don't want to hear more about why they should feed, but how.

In the first few months of life, the time it takes to nurse a baby is equivalent to an 8- to 9-hour workday for most women. Most babies will drain a breast in about 12 to 15 minutes if they are eager and actively feeding, but babies often stay on the breast for up to 20 or even 30 minutes at a time. Therefore, if you sit down, feed your baby on the right, feed your baby on the left, burp the baby, and change the inevitable diaper—poof, 1 hour. And most newborns feed up to 8 to 10 times daily. 1 + 1 + 1 + 1 + 1 + 1 + 1 + 1 + 1. Math is easy when you do it this way. Breastfeeding alone is a full-time job for the first few months.

Therefore, mothers who go back to work early in their newborns' lives are really tackling the challenges of a few jobs: the mom job, the milk supplier, and the worker bee. Challenge, yes. Surmountable, of course, but this study points out some flaws in our expectation of the singular worker-bee/milk-supplier/momma person.

- Women were less likely to continue breastfeeding if they went back to work before 12 weeks (the average for all women in the study was return to work at 10 weeks).
- Stress level and position at work (if inflexible or not a supervisor level) affect women's ability to continue breastfeeding. In my experience and in the experience of my patients, I've found this to be true again and again.
- Women with maternity leave for fewer than or equal to 6 weeks had a 3-fold increased risk of quitting breastfeeding compared with moms who didn't return to work.

Cessation of breastfeeding can be traumatic for all involved. While 45 states in the United States have laws relating to breastfeeding, only 28 states have laws that exempt breastfeeding from public indecency laws. Shockingly, only 24 states have laws related to women in the workplace. Therefore, it can be diffi-cult for women to protect breastfeeding goals once back at work, and where you live may change this reality. The benefits from breastfeeding are astound-ing. Pediatricians work hard to support families in their goals to breastfeed their babies, knowing well that the benefits are worth the initial struggles.

Maternal-baby bonding, reduced stomach infections, reduced ear infections, reduced rates of obesity, and reduced hospitalizations are just a few of the benefits to breastfeeding infants. Moms who choose to breastfeed and work and find success at doing both, simultaneously, amaze. They expect great things of themselves. And although they should expect great things of themselves, the stresses of attending a job, caring for a newborn, and supporting their own bodies with good nutrition, hydration, and rest to make breast milk may at times be Herculean.

Tips for Successful Transitions Back to Work While Breastfeeding

- Make a plan for breastfeeding before you have the baby. Ah, yes, yet another to-do for your list. Do this. Discuss with coworkers, supervisors, your boss, or anyone else at work who is experienced where and how they suggest you find time in your workday and a safe, clean place to breastfeed or pump breast milk when you return to work. Do this before you leave. You'll shape expectations.
- Rally your troops. Tell your spouse, partner, or good friends (in and out of work) your goals for breastfeeding and ask for their help during your transition back to work (meals, phone calls, texting while attached to the pump, magazines to read).
- Have patience with yourself if some days your milk production is down. Stress, dehydration, illness, separation from the baby, and pumping versus feeding can all affect your milk supply. If you only pump 2 ounces on Tuesday at work, don't give up! You never know what Wednesday can bring…
- Partial breastfeeding is better than no breastfeeding. Most policy statements and studies compare exclusive breastfeeding to no breastfeeding. Often I hear a paternalistic, disappointing tone from advocates for breastfeeding. And mom after mom tells me that it intimidates them. The reality is that many babies receive a safe mix of breast milk and formula during the first year. If you find you have to supplement your infant once you or your partner is back to work, fine! Formula is good for babies too. Unload the guilt as best you can. After your baby drinks the pumped breast milk, have your partner or child care provider offer formula if you think the supply of milk from pumping is down in the mother's absence.
- The availability of work-site lactation facilities is well known to affect breastfeeding success. If you're not comfortable with the spot you have been

offered for pumping breast milk, ask for another. A clean, private, lockable non-bathroom location to express milk is the law of the land (see "Mama Doc Vitals" below). There is nothing less conducive to pumping milk than a scary, unclean, unlocked, cold, exposed, or intimidating place. It is never too late to ask. It is OK to revisit this issue even if you've found yourself pumping milk in the walk-in refrigerator at work for a month. If need be, make a phone call to talk to the supervisor of your supervisor if it can help decrease the tension for you having to ask directly in the workplace.

- Do the ridiculous. Fill your pumping bag with photos of your baby. Carry a water bottle everywhere you go. Take the break you need to go and pump milk even when inconvenient to the needs of your work. Leave work on time. Continue to take your prenatal vitamins so the milk you make doesn't deplete you.
- Then be easy on yourself or your partner, who is trying to do it all. If you can't do it, you can't do it. Find support in others' experiences. Talk to your friends and you'll find you have many allies in these waters.
- Make reasonable, short-term breastfeeding goals. Instead of thinking to yourself every day, "I have to make it to 9 months," think to yourself, "I am going to try my best to breastfeed until 4:00 pm tomorrow." When 4:00 pm tomorrow comes, pick a new target. This tactic helped me prolong my pumping months.
- As best you can, be kind to yourself on the days this is a challenge. Your baby is so lucky to have you this committed to her health and nutrition!

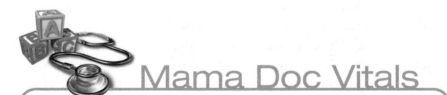

Mama Doc Vitals

Tip: A clean, private, lockable non-bathroom location to express milk is the law of the land: US Department of Labor: http://bit.ly/mdm-NursingMothers.

Breastfeeding Laws: http://bit.ly/mdm-BreastfeedingLaws

Families Resource Guide: http://bit.ly/mdm-BreastfeedingResources

79

Complex Problem: Raising a Child

I had the fortune of seeing Atul Gawande, MD, MPH, speak in Seattle. Truth be told, I entirely invited myself. I heard there was a group from the hospital going and I begged my way in. I sat in the corner. Flashbacks to finding a seat in the junior high cafeteria. I made it through the seating time and forgot all about the awkward act of my self-inviting and seat-finding by the end. Despite my disrespect for Ms Manners and my loud mouth, my pushy ways afforded me the opportunity to witness a leader in medicine.

I enjoyed what Dr Gawande said about his work in using checklists to ultimately decrease complications and death in the surgical setting. I have read Dr Gawande's books (or parts of them, I admit) and many of his articles in *The New Yorker* (whole thing, thank you). I marvel at his skill and ease of writing, his ability to translate complicated problems and make you feel like you thought of them yourself due to their apparent simplicity. His assertions, however, are not simple. It's just that his skill in expressing his position, explaining the breakdowns in the system, and offering opinions wed with solution puts us all at ease. His article, "The Cost Conundrum," remains one of my favorite articles of all time. I have read it numerous times and think about it when caring for children on a weekly basis. He has affirmed the way I feel about over-testing in medicine. As I have said previously, in pediatrics, so often, less is more.

When he spoke in Seattle he used a metaphor that delighted me. When he said it, a grin appeared on my face. One of those grins you have when you know you belong or feel included in an elite group. In this case, the group is parents. I was reminded of my good luck and good fortune in being a mom. His mention of it demonstrates the simple brilliance I have seen in Dr Gawande's words before. After his talk he took questions from the audience, which was a mix of physicians, business and health care workers, and administrators. In discussing some differences in medical problems, he categorized as follows:

- **There are simple problems,** like making a cake and following the directions on the box.
- **There are complicated problems,** like launching and preparing a rocket ship for a trip to the moon.
- **And then there are complex problems,** like raising a child.

  Enough said, Dr Gawande. Thanks for the affirmation.

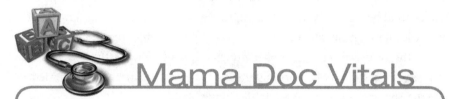

Article: "The Cost Conundrum: What a Texas Town Can Teach Us About Health Care": http://bit.ly/mdm-CostConundrum

Nothing I Learned in Medical School: On Parenting

I stumbled on an article summary online recently: "Bad Behavior Linked to Poor Parenting." I am going to call this BBLtPP. I clicked on the link with butterflies, hoping not to find something like, "We're following a pediatrician with 2 sons, one doctor husband, and one overweight Labrador who live in Seattle. She writes a blog. It's her parenting we're worried about...." But I clicked on the link and it didn't exist; I got an error message. Then again, nothing. Clicked a few minutes later. Nothing. The page on MSNBC, for some reason, had vanished.

Thank goodness.

I hate seeing reports like this in the media. They propel this myth that there is one way to do this, this raising of child. When *American Idol* advertised for "Mom Idol" on television, I wondered, was Mom Idol going to sing or just win for being the best all-around rock-and-roll mom? I'm certain not to win in both categories. I'm sure I'm doing something wrong. Parent-teacher preschool conference next week, so I'll let you know. But really, what defines ideal mother-hood, and who is the one doing the defining?

The immense task and joy of raising, loving, feeding, and enriching a child's life while gaining incredible perspective along the way seems utterly undefinable at times. Articles like BBLtPP strike deep stomach drops and fear in many of us. I know this. My patients tell me about these types of articles. Then they ask questions like, "Do you feel it's wrong if I give her peaches before avocados?" Seemingly basic question, but it's loaded with self-doubt. There is a particular look in their eyes. It's, "I'm a bad parent, aren't I?" But their mouth forms the words "a-v-o-c-a-d-o" and "p-e-a-c-h-e-s."

This idea that there is a right way and a wrong way to parent is nothing I learned in medical school or pediatric residency. Rather, it's something I've learned at the mommy group I went to a few times, or the playground I visit, or the snide comments I got while feeding my son a bottle of formula in Seattle. The limited and rigorous idea that there is an essentially scripted good way versus bad way to parent needs no further emphasis in the media.

There are safety concerns and gross errors in parenting. I'm not entirely naive, of course. I have cared for many children who are the victims of the lack of parenting—assaulted children, abused children, abandoned and neglected ones. I am not saying that there are no lines in this sand. There really are right (evidence and lifesaving) ways to have your baby sleep, safer ways to feed and avoid choking, safer ways to play, and safer ways to protect and buckle your child into a car. But those tasks and preventive measures for preserving and promoting health aren't the essence of parenting.

Parenting is all the other things in between.

The mortar, really. The sticky stuff wedged between all the tasks and lists we check off throughout the day and night with our children. At the risk of sounding all Hallmark, I'd say it's the really good stuff. Parenting is the consistency, the listening, the remembering. The unconditional love part. Parenting comes when you enjoy or laugh with your child, when you respond to their cry, when you remember who they are and how to help them regain their idea of themselves. It's when you advocate for them in difficult situations. Or in easy ones. When you provide them a trusted and reliable model and space to be. When you provide them a platform to grow and develop. Parenting is grossly individual.

I watch parenting happen every day when I'm in clinic. And at home. It happens all the time. But I still don't have a manual.

My sons are growing me up too. Just as they gain inches and pounds, I gain insight, wisdom, and conscience for the world.

Most of us perform constant self-evaluation. The ubiquitous running monologue. "Am I doing this right? Am I a bad parent if I _____?" Rarely, I suppose the answer is yes. More often, no.

We constantly self-monitor, self-reflect, and project ourselves against our peers and family, coworkers, and neighbors.

Oh, crud. Just tried the BBLtPP link again and it goes through when you hit refresh. The first sentence reads, "Poor parenting causes boys, but few girls, to be particularly prone to bad behavior, a new study suggests."

Now it's stacked against me! Good grief. You read it if you'd like, but I don't think I'll pick apart the study for you. Instincts on my back, I believe the 4 of us will find our way in this house. Mom Idol or not, with help from my dear friends and family, I'll hopefully avoid showing up in the study labeled "bad parent" while Finn and Oden grow me up too.

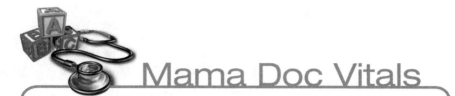

Link: "Bad behavior linked to poor parenting" article on NBC News Web site: http://bit.ly/mdm-behavior

81

Four Hours on a School Bus

So many of my patients have food allergies, as do many children of my friends. With food allergies now affecting 1 in 13 children, most every classroom has a child at risk. It's life that has taught me the complex stew of worry, hope, and diligence that comes together for parents who support and feed a child with severe allergies. The stories I hear and parents I learn from have really changed how I help support children in my practice and community.

A good friend wrote a "secret, imaginary blog post" and sent it my way. I realized instantly it was a *real* blog post. But to protect her son and allow the imaginary (blog) to become real, she called on her childhood and the beloved author Judy Blume for help. She chose the pen name Veronica.

Then Nancy decided we should all have secret sensational names such as Alexandra, Veronica, Kimberly, and Mavis. Nancy got to be Alexandra. I was Mavis.
—*Are You There God? It's Me, Margaret* by Judy Blume

"Veronica" is an awesome friend, a passionate researcher, and mom of 2. Like all of us, she has stumbled on unexpected challenges in protecting her children from harm. In particular, protecting her son with severe food allergies. Her writing helped me see more clearly what it is like to love, care for, and support a child with severe and life-threatening food allergies. What it is like to wave good-bye for a day of school…and house worry inside your chest. And really, what it is like to have no choice but to go well out of the way.

Four Hours on a School Bus: Parenting and Severe Food Allergies
By Veronica Z

Four hours on a school bus. Because I go on every field trip. Because none of the teachers is certified to give my child his lifesaving medication if he needs it. And yet he won't need it today. But he might. And so I sit on a school bus for 4 hours. Bouncing along with screaming kids, singing kids, sleeping kids. My own kid sitting with his friends at the back of the bus while I sit in the middle of the bus, supervising other kids. Because he no longer needs me. Or no longer needs to sit with me, anyway. But I need him. I need him to live. I need to guard against every preventable accident. I need to think ahead to every holiday party, birthday party, unexpected celebration, and field trip. No matter how far into the countryside. No matter that there will be no threat to him today. No outside food. No unexpected snack. No candy snuck onto the bus by another kid. No reason for me to be there. Except that I'm a food allergy mom. I'm always there. The Zelig of preschool, pre-K, K, first grade, second grade. Room parent at the ready. Volunteering for every occasion when my child may encounter an allergen. Because I want him to live. And I don't want him to worry too much. And I don't want to be too much trouble to the teacher. And I don't want to make too big deal out of this. But I do want my child to live. Four hours on a school bus today. That was our food allergy tax. It was a high tariff, but I paid it. Turns out I didn't need to. But I didn't know that this morning. I never know until it's over. So I pay it every time. Every. Time.

There are silver linings. I "get" to go on as many pumpkin patch, museum, or musical theater trips as I can manage. I know the birthday of every kid in the classroom. I bring a homemade cupcake, like an offering, to every party. But it's not for the birthday kid. It's for my kid. I'm paying the food allergy tax. No store-bought shortcuts. It's some other kid's birthday, but I'm baking. I'm baking a whole batch of cupcakes so my kid has one safe one.

Here's what I tell new acquaintances: Imagine a life with no takeout, no last-minute meal plans, no "Hey, let's just order pizza" or "Let's go out to eat." We cook from scratch. We know the ingredients of everything we have in the house. It changes the way you eat. It makes you lose patience when a list of ingredients takes a long time to read. So you stick with less-processed food. Unless it's Oreos. Because those are awesome. Shelf-stable sugar for those occasions when all your plans are for nothing. Someone decides that today is the day they are bringing in cupcakes. I'm out of town or out of flour, or sugar, or vegetable oil. No cupcakes in the freezer. Oreos to the rescue.

WendySueSwanson MD @SeattleMamaDoc

Good grief, kids can be mean. This is news to me: 1/3 of kids with food allergies are teased/bullied at school http://bit.ly/bz7M6M

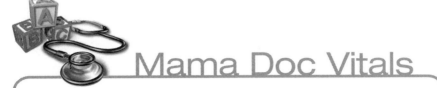

Mama Doc Vitals

Link: Kids With Food Allergies: http://bit.ly/mdm-FoodAllergies

Tip: For babies starting on solids: introduce the same food daily for a day or two. Give your baby a chance to explore the new texture and flavor. Then 3 days later, add on another new food. That way in the rare case of an allergy or intolerance, you'll know what food to blame.

Study: A 2013 study in *The Journal of Allergy and Clinical Immunology* (http://bit.ly/mdm-AllergyPrevent) found that adding wheat, rye, oats, and barley before 5½ months, fish before 9 months, and egg before 11 months was associated with lower rates of asthma, allergic rhinitis, and allergic response in the blood.

Tip: It's no longer recommended to wait on introduction of "allergic" food. Introducing egg, peanuts, fish, and wheat prior to 1 year of age is recommended.

82

When Parenthood Exceeds Expectations

We surfaced, my husband and me. Bobbed up after having been submerged in the challenges and complexities of stress, tantrums, hectic schedules, holiday crunch time, and career responsibilities. When we surfaced, we found ourselves in one of the most luxurious moments of life. It was one of those spells I want to compound. More than just burning it on my brain, I want to relive that memory again and again. I want to hit play and repeat…I suppose that's part of why I'm sharing it here.

Here's what I mean. Have you had one of those meals or nights or walks or adventures with your children recently where you realize there is simply nothing better? Where you wake up in a moment and consider that it is for this moment, this one space in the continuum of time, that you were made to be? When you come to feel like it's why you're alive?

In my opinion, it happens to all of us in profoundly new ways when we are lucky enough to raise children. And it's usually unexpected. These pristine, magical moments with our children and family don't come with proper planning. They don't usually happen on vacation, at the fancy meal, or at the picnic we've planned for 2 weeks. We often don't have our fancy shoes on. The moments tumble into our lives when we least expect it with absolutely zero material value. But like falling in love for the first time, these moments sweep us up off our feet and arrive without a hint of warning.

This is, I believe, the gift of the season of our lives. When parenthood exceeds expectations.

Recently, I was talking with a good friend about these rare moments. The ones that happen when your children are enticed by conversation, fully engaged in a game or meal, when they get along with each other, and you realize there is nothing more precious or intimate. Often it seems that these moments follow illness or fear. But sometimes it doesn't take a trigger or challenge. Recently, a moment appeared for my friend when she and her husband had cancelled a date night. They were too exhausted and decided to stay home and have dinner with their children and just crash. And it happened—the moment—they connected, their children were angels at dinner, delighted and laughing, present and mindful. She and her husband looked up at each other and realized they were woven into one of those meals they wouldn't trade the world for. Really.

For us it happened late Thursday night on the floor of our living room. Our 6-year-old had received Mastermind (a board game) for his birthday and the 4 of us teamed up to play. It was the first time I'd played in 25 years and each of us approached the game with excitement. We were enticed to win, eager, and we each giggled as we navigated and explored ways to outsmart the others.

And there we were, lying on a hard wooden floor, surrounded by the darkness of winter, entirely together with only little plastic playing pieces between us. Momentous connection and family intimacy. I can barely articulate why and how I knew it was one of those moments except that I realized this is really *as good as it gets*.

83

"Having It All": Stumbling

I read the 2012 *Atlantic* piece written by Anne-Marie Slaughter entitled, "Why Women Still Can't Have It All." Make sure you block off a half day from work if you want to read it. It takes a good number of minutes to get through, and I found myself kind of staring at the wall after I'd finished. Slaughter does a beautiful job spelling out the glaring issues of our time for working women using her intense personal experience and her extensive education. She lays out her thesis for our inability to "have it all" as working mothers circa 2012, and she illuminates the traps so many of us stumble into as we work and raise our children. Yet knowing all this didn't really help in the immediate.

Differing gender roles, division of responsibility issues at home, and the juggle (tug-of-war) many women feel with balancing the needs of their family and the needs of their careers aren't new. But Ms Slaughter does draw us in. I haven't had a chance to chat about it at any water cooler, but I have watched and listened and lingered online. The article was a huge success for the magazine; even my husband notices a dust cloud at work. A ripple in the lake of life for many of us, for sure.

Let me break down my response in a few chunks. This isn't exactly steady and linear for me. This isn't a thesis or rebuttal, just a reaction.

No One Has It All; We're All Missing Out on Something

I don't think, "I've got it all." I'm not certain I've met anyone who does. At least, I don't think they have it all, all in one moment. I do, however, have a career in medicine, 2 thrilling children, a thriving partnership with my husband, a dream to make change in the world, rich supportive friendships, and an overweight Labrador. Some days I don't have time to eat enough; some days I do. Some days the stress is sky-high; some days it isn't. Some days I laugh a lot and pause to absorb the moment. Some days I work more than 15 hours. Some days I'm filled with a shivering mindfulness while in the midst of my boys. Some days I can't imagine being anywhere else but in the examination room with my patients. Some days I can.

The discomfort for me is that when I'm away from my children, I am always less whole. Their needs continue to shift, the work-life balance target moves, and all the while the distance from them remains apparent. It's always easier for me to exist when my boys are only paces away. This is the hefty reality of parenthood that begins on day one.

Slaughter points out that this experience can be very different for women and men. And this could be very different if our society supported our dual roles better.

Even so, the concept of "having it all" gets distorted at the virtual water cooler as we're urged to think about what we're missing somewhere. If we're educated and have skills to work, the minute our children are born we're set up to miss out on *something*. And it can be torture in moments for stay-at-home mom (SAHM) or working mom. It's the opportunities that wait for us in our work or the time at home with our children; someone will always tell us we're missing something.

This conversation is one that comes only with the privilege of choice (with work), anyway.

Regardless, it's women who are still set up to do the heavy lifting in these conversations. I know men do too. But in my experience (like Slaughter's), it's women who are suffering in these choices. Our stake in the conversation starts early for most of us—a pregnancy followed by a (short) maternity leave— people start to ask us about where we'll "be" after the baby's born, and in my experience, that question never stops being asked.

Women still make around 70 cents on the dollar for the same work. And studies have found that women physicians, for example, may make less money because they choose to spend more time with their patients. So it may be that we working women want something different, rather than "it all." One take-home from Slaughter's article for me was that I don't think I want it all—it's not the goal. I want to use what I've been given, soak up the gift of my children, and give back all I can. I want to enjoy the choices I make; articles like Slaughter's tend to take me away from that.

The Stumble

I certainly still stumble, believing that others may "have it all" or that I should want it. I'll meet a mom who will tell me she is working the "perfect amount." Or a colleague/peer/friend/family member will tell me about a mother who is delighted to report that she quit her job and finds herself on a Tuesday in the park with her children. In these stories, this mother inevitably looks up to the sky and realizes, "It's perfect." When I hear these parenting tales, my stomach will drop, I'll get a little shiver, or I'll worry I'm in the wrong spot at the wrong time (in life). And I stumble.

I also stumbled as I bid farewell to a coworker who left her job at our clinic to be with her children for the summer. She plans to find a job where her work schedule shadows her children's schedule. And while I witnessed her struggle to leave a job she loved, I also saw her make the brave choice to make change; it all seemed so entirely sensible, so smart, and so centered. Stumble.

I stumble believing that another working woman's equation or theory (Slaughter's, for example) may illuminate my perfect equation for balance and personal/professional success. Trouble is, no one parent has the same set of circumstances, the same set of goals, the same set of education, the same set of skills, and the same children and partner as another. The lives we create are fingerprints—entirely unique.

All these rocks in the road that cause us to veer off path never weigh exactly the same as our own core. And so we continue to stumble.

Cloning

I often return to the one solution I've come up with when it comes to "having it all" or striking perfection with long-lasting balance. Cloning. If I could just have a few of me, I could be simultaneously caring for patients in clinic, exploring the planet with my boys, communicating health stories to the public, and providing self-care (exercise, good healthy meals, rest, reflection, and relaxation). I could live diversely all the time for all those who count on me and chart the path I most want as well. Maybe then I'd really have it all.

Of course, my neurotic solution is a ludicrous retort to the menacing problem the *Atlantic* article hones in on: the quest for happiness and balance among highly educated parents working and living chaotic lives with their children. And that's the real lesson, I suppose. Perfection on the working/parenting fulcrum simply won't and doesn't exist for any of us. We may have to flush out our goals for happiness before we distill the path to perfection—and we may have to act like humans. We may just need to get up each day open to the possibility of enjoying it, changing it, and witnessing it. And some days, that must be more than enough—even for we working moms.

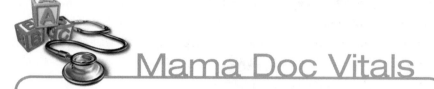

Mama Doc Vitals

Slaughter's Article: http://bit.ly/mdm-WorkingMoms

Responses: "Men Never 'Had It All'" (http://bit.ly/mdm-WorkingDads); "Can Women Have It All?" (http://bit.ly/mdm-HavingItAll); "Mothers: Don't Lie to Your Employers When You Do Kid Things During the Day" (http://bit.ly/mdm-KidThings)

"The Retro Wife": http://bit.ly/mdm-RetroWife

84

The Tiger Mom

I've read more than 40 to 50 reviews of the Tiger Mom and her book. If for some reason you've not heard of her (Who are you? They're looking for you to sit on a jury somewhere), Amy Chua is a self-declared Tiger Mom. She wrote a piece entitled, "Why Chinese Mothers are Superior," in *The Wall Street Journal* January 8, 2011. It marks the beginning of the Amy Chua era. Since then, buzz around her book, *Battle Hymn of the Tiger Mother,* persists. I still hear moms mention "the Tiger Mom" in clinic.

I didn't want to write about Tiger Mom and the media frenzy that ensued when her book came out. I didn't want to lend credit to her media bonanza. And truthfully, I've been intimidated by the exceptional writing in response to her biting words. At first, I didn't think I had anything unique to add. I don't like her message (tough/conditional love, tyranny and insults, achievement = happiness), but she probably doesn't like mine either. I have high expectations for myself, my friends, my family, and my coworkers. I expect my children to challenge themselves, learn to communicate, learn to love, and work hard to make their conditions good enough so they can enjoy their lives. *I expect them to contribute.* I may roar, but I really don't bite. I don't hit, spank, grab, or insult either. I expect, at particular points in life, that many people won't meet my expectations, just like I won't meet theirs. I believe in forgiveness. My love and adoration doesn't waver based on performance.

We don't tolerate aggression in our children; why would we tolerate it in ourselves? Abuse is far more complicated than that which comes from the force of a fist. Just to be clear, I'll never call my children, "Garbage."

I don't want to read her book. The more I read about her, the less I want to know about what she says. I'd rather read something by Peggy Orenstein. I do, however, remain drawn to read what other people think about what this Tiger says. There is an unequivocal sociology brewing. Clearly Amy Chua did more than strike a chord. What's interesting is not Chua's idea (that one privileged, hyper-educated, heavily connected, wealthy, Chinese American mom believes her parenting is superior), but rather the response of our nation. I mean, everyone has something to say about this. Why would we care that some mom, in one corner of our country, thinks she is doing a better job raising her kids? Why would we care that she equates happiness with achievement or "Westerners" with weakness? Why would we care that she believes intellect is only captured in music capability/competitions and SAT scores? She misses so much about humanity. So much about what defines our connection to others. We care, I suspect, because she was strong enough to state that she believed she was right. And that she's better.

She's a bully. And a lucky one. Her kids have the wealth of good health.

Read the most memorable response I've read, to keep any fascination with Amy Chua's words in check.

Battle Hymn of a Bereaved Mother
by Carin Towne

During the past couple weeks it seems Amy Chua and the promotion of her book "Battle Hymn of the Tiger Mother" are everywhere – The Wall Street Journal, The New York Times, The Seattle Times, Time, and even in my People Magazine. Somehow I have managed to let the premise of her narrative get under my skin, which I'm pretty sure is her intention. A disclaimer: I have not read her book. But I have read enough excerpts now to be reminded of how different my life is from hers. It is becoming increasingly clear to me that in a world of parenting books and philosophies – how to raise your children right, discipline the right way, how to maximize your child's potential, and more – those "right ways" no longer fit for our family. For they assume that a) your child does not have special needs mentally or physically and that b) your child does not get cancer and die.

Prior to Ben's illness, I could have been accused of trying to parent the "right" or perfect way. I had an ever-growing library of "how to" books. But Ben's diagnosis blew everything out of the water. Watching him suffer beyond my worst imagination and die in front of me has, needless to say, completely changed me as a person and parent. Ryan now has, for better or worse, a different mom. My goals for him are very simple: live. Surely, I want him to be a positive contributing member of society. I hope he goes to college. But my expectations are vastly different from Ms. Chua's. Am I a Westernized parent? Or a golden retriever mom? Perhaps. Or maybe I am just a bereaved mom, who has been forced to recognize that life can change in one second and ultimately our children's lives are not in our control.

Yet, in what I can control, I know this to be true: I want Ryan to be happy, to do something he finds joy in, to love and be loved. The rest is up for grabs. I could care less if he becomes a musical prodigy or goes to Harvard. Of course if one of those happens because of his own dreams I will be immensely proud of him. But his success, or lack of success, in terms of worldly judgment means little to me. I will not be crazed if he doesn't practice violin for three hours a day, nor deny him food under any circumstances. That's what happens when your first child is fed through a nose tube. The only thing at this point that I can think of that will be my undoing is if he threatens his own life in any way. If he does something stupid that verges on a reunion with his brother I will bring my wrath down faster than the humidity in New Jersey can ruin my straightened hair. But I guarantee you I will never tell my son he is "garbage". And I doubt that word would come to mind again for Ms. Chua in reference to her daughter if she saw her hooked up to oxygen, unconscious and days away from death.

Do we watch too much TV in our house for brain development experts – probably. Do we jump on the bed more than other families? I am guessing yes. Do I give him – within reason – what he likes to eat? I do. Does Ryan still receive time outs? Of course! I want people to like him. Do I let him do whatever his little three year old crazy brain desires while praising him incessantly and imagining rainbows and butterflies dancing over his head? Of course not. But there are not a lot of "rights" anymore. There are just the three of us, trying to do the best we can each day – without the other member of our family. And while I in no way, shape or form would ever wish Ms. Chua's daughters, or anyone, to be diagnosed with a life threatening illness – I do wish people like her could live in my shoes for a moment. For in doing so, my guess is they would be a little less self-righteous about the way they parent and perhaps for a minute they would love their child for who they are instead of who they want them to become. For if I had only loved Ben for whom he would have become I would have been severely disappointed.

I'll tell you, I won plenty of music competitions (oboe), I went to an Ivy league medical school, I have a good job and an innovative career, I married a fantastic partner, and I have the fortune of raising 2 darling boys. I didn't come anywhere close to perfecting the SATs, I made mistakes, I quit lots of things along the way. Clearly I don't think my accomplishments (or failures) define my worth, my happiness, or my sense of purpose. I agree more with David Brooks when he said, "Amy Chua Is a Wimp." Brooks points out that, "Practicing a piece of music for four hours requires focused attention, but it is nowhere near as cognitively demanding as a sleepover with 14-year-old girls." Emotional intellect means something. We test for it, just not inside the classroom. And it's far more difficult to measure than math.

I didn't grow up with a Tiger Mom; my mom was more of a lion. There was a roar and an expectation, a sense of doing for myself, a sense of owning actions and responsibility. But no ultimate conditions, per se. No insults. My parents didn't pay me (or punish me) for grades. I could get what I wanted out of school, they said. My family believed it should come from me. As a colleague wrote, "Self-discipline comes from within." My lion-mom had lines in the sand, yes. But she watched and listened for preferences and for explanations too. It seemed to work.

As do a bagillion other parenting styles.

Tiger Mom's book feels calculated and corrupt, borrowing time and energy from a nation that doubts itself. A parenting book gowned as a "memoir," I believe her book was written in part to sell and to stir.

Ultimately It Comes Down to This

Constant self-evaluation is an unfortunate part of parenthood for most of us. Thanks to the accessibility of information online, the mommy blogosphere, the rise of social media, ongoing traditional media, Aunt Jane and her opinions alongside mother-in-law Trudy, we know what everybody thinks about pacifiers and breastfeeding, antibiotics or BPA, our strategies for getting our baby to sleep, and our choice of sports for our children. Everyone seems to have an opinion when it comes to raising our children. Everyone, at one time or another, feels they are *right*. They likely are. But within seconds online, we can get to places where others disagree with what we're doing. Devoutly. We can immediately distrust our instincts and our choices.

What a lovely world in which to raise a child.

But we go looking. Don't we? Late at night, between feedings, before work, or while pumping. Parents are online every day searching for health and parenting information, community, and fellowship. I believe this search is defined, in large part, by a quest for camaraderie, not fulfillment of any self-loathing. The big issue that makes us want to talk about Chua is that the results to our searches online may lead us astray. We may be left feeling deficient instead of steadied. After reading a blog post, a parenting manual, or a memoir, we often come to distrust.

This is why Chua stuck a Carnegie-Hall–type chord.

Amy Chua has backtracked since the *Wall Street Journal* piece, stating that her book isn't a parenting book but a memoir. I've read that she didn't have final say on the title of the piece in the *Wall Street Journal.* I've read that she wouldn't have entitled her methods, "Superior." But that seems an odd rebuttal, particularly for someone who aims and excels in perfection.

Being socially connected is profoundly important to happiness. Enjoying our parenthood is too.

I think what we really need to ask ourselves, post-Tiger Mom, is when will we love the parent we are today?

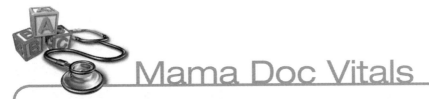

Mama Doc Vitals

Carin Towne graciously allowed me to include her blog post in the book. Please consider visiting her foundation Web site, www.bentownefoundation.org, to learn more about Carin and Jeff's foundation in honor of their son, The Ben Towne Pediatric Cancer Research Foundation.

More About Ben: Benjamin Ward Towne was born on July 17, 2005, to parents Jeff and Carin Towne. He was a fiercely determined, passionate, and loving little boy. Ben enjoyed cars, tennis, golf, the beach, and his family. In August 2007, just a month after his second birthday, Ben was diagnosed with stage 4 high-risk neuroblastoma. His only presenting symptom was a discoloration around his eyes. Treatment included 6 courses of chemotherapy, surgery, stem cell transplant, radiation, 5 rounds of antibody therapy, and more. Ben was in remission in July 2008, only to relapse catastrophically in October. He died on December 30, 2008.

Ben's parents have taken this incredibly challenging journey and committed to improving the lives of others. Astonishing, really.

"The Wife"

One little thing that really gets under my skin, if you must know, is the title, "The Wife." When I hear it, it rings through me, moving and shifting my electrons in just the wrong way.

I'm sure most of you wives or mothers out there on planet Earth don't really mind it. But I do.

Here is how I often hear it. Let me set the scene.

Examination room, child center stage, father stage left. Meaning no harm (or disrespect), the dad says, "Oh, and *the wife* wanted me to ask you about this rash."

I remain calm, usually leaking no erratic response, remark, or expression. This is my issue, I'm sure. But the internal alarm goes off. Just something about that woman being distilled to "the wife."

"My wife wanted me to ask you about this rash." No alarm.

"His mother wanted me to ask you about this rash." No alarm.

But, "The wife wanted me to ask you about this rash." Alarm-tastic.

With permission, I'm going to refer to my partner and husband, father of my children, as *The Husband*. Just to even the field. For today and maybe tomorrow too. He's OK with it; I've cleared this.

Thank you, The Husband.

Magic

Sometimes good health feels like magic. Lately more than ever. I've had a number of friends and family diagnosed with serious medical problems and medical setbacks. Like patients that I have been fortunate enough to care for with serious illness, it scares me, makes me sad, sometimes wakes me up at night. These episodes in illness are disorienting to the order of things. These diagnoses, uncertainties, and realities are especially weighty in December amid bags of gifts, holiday music, lit trees, and piped-in joy. Fear amid cheer. Ultimately, these diagnoses and fears feel really real and make the rest of life blur. I suppose I just feel more angular, vulnerable, and then compassionate right now. Ever aware of the good health that surrounds me too. Perspective defined.

When I was getting my tooth drilled (horrifying, really, having someone drill your tooth, yes?) I didn't even really flinch. Even though I am absurdly scared of the dentist. See, this newfound perspective of feeling healthy, lucky, and fortunate amid some who aren't, is clarifying. The zoom-out, zoom-in of life. When we see and know clearly how absolutely good it is to feel well.

But then, there has been some magic too. When my first son was just 3 years old, he fell and cut up his hand badly. He required stiches in the emergency department. And when I look back at that scar and his hand back together, functional, beautiful—it's magic. Skin healing is magic.

And then more magic. I don't know what happened, which stars crossed, or how the winds blew in the right direction, but the day my second started to walk felt magical. He took about 6 steps toward me one night while on vacation. And of course, then did it again. By the end of the evening, he was covered in sweat like a professional boxer. He was battling his milestone and winning. Gowned in pride, crossing the room. My favorite milestone, I have no idea why, happened again. My little baby turned big boy and walked across the room.

Then magic happened again when my oldest wore underwear for the first time. You know how pediatricians often talk about toilet training happening somewhere between age 2 and 3 years? Well, Finn has blown past those dates.

Imagine him running and looking back over his shoulder at 3, laughing. But on the very day this past week that Oden started to walk, Finn donned his underwear, inspired by his older cousin.

Walking, underwear, healing, and skin. Magic.

Now cross your toes that my friend with her newly diagnosed cancer, my 2 family members who have spent too much time at the doctor, and all those lovely, brave people out there who are hurting uncover magic too.

87

Open Letter to Marissa Mayer

I started to see a number of tweets from parents and fellow pediatricians on Twitter criticizing Marissa Mayer for announcing that she'd return to work within 1 to 2 weeks of the delivery of her first child.

First off, I'll start with my assumptions.

I'm in the belief that Ms Mayer has access to quality health care; that is, she has the ear of a board-certified obstetrician and a board-certified pediatrician and access to a lactation consultant as needed. My hunch is that if she needs information on evidence-based ramifications, from a health perspective, of going back to work 1 to 2 weeks postpartum, she can get the data she needs. Because she used to work at Google, I suspect she understands how to find what she needs online as well.

Assumptions acknowledged, I'd like to give Ms Mayer the respect she deserves. Faulting her for not making a traditional choice is devoid of context. She is lauded for her enormously successful career at a young age. She is the youngest CEO of any Fortune 500 company. To me it appears she has savvy and skill, invention, and grit. Thanks in part to Ms Mayer as the first female engineer at Google, we enjoy an entirely different electronic world with Gmail, Google search, maps, and images.

As we expect and work to have women hold an increased share of leadership jobs, academic or not, we must acknowledge that we can't have it both ways. We can't want and wait for more and more women to have their hands at the wheels of powerful companies and organizations, only to question their commitment to their personal and children's health and well-being when they return to work. One week or 6 months postpartum.

I suspect Ms Mayer is making decisions in the context of what is right for her family. Her job security and her value in moving her company forward are a part of that. We make good decisions when we reflect on all those who are affected by our actions. Only we know how to prioritize our choices. I've yet to hear what her husband plans for the upcoming months. It's possible he'll be at the beck and call of this new baby. Why do we so often forget the realities of shared parenting?

Further, this discussion misses a very important reality. Many of the new moms I get to see in clinic don't work outside their homes. Women who work in their homes raising children often return to work within days of delivering a child. Stay-at-home moms often come to the clinic 3-day postpartum visit alone with 2 to 4 children in tow. This reality reflects the stay-at-home mom commitment to career too.

The banter continued as Ms Mayer was criticized for using crowdsourcing to name her child. I remain jaw-dropped that we could find another reason to fault her savvy, her nimble skill with technology, and assault her again as she begins the journey of motherhood.

The beautiful thing is this: None of us get access to the intimate bond she and her child will develop and cherish with their time together on Earth. *I also suspect she's not looking for advice.*

Congratulations, Marissa Mayer. It's my hope that you delighted in the most precious transition imaginable. That you had the time and space to inhale the health and vitality of your new baby amid your growing family. I am in awe of what you do for us all. And I trust you to make phenomenal decisions for your son.

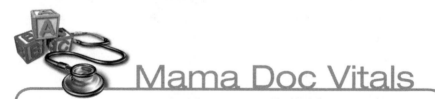

Mama Doc Vitals

Blog Post: "Women Still Missing From Medicine's Top Ranks" by Danielle Ofri, MD: http://bit.ly/mdm-TopRanks

Tip: The perfect "balance" with work and children is a moving target. One lesson I've learned from my clinical practice: don't ever underestimate your power to redesign how you work.

One Mother's Day Gift

I already got my Mother's Day gift for the decade. It came in 2 parts and it only cost $25.

It started on a Wednesday. I had an over-scheduled day of meetings, my mom's chemotherapy, a luncheon (that I ended up not making), blog stuff, patient calls, and an interview for local PBS. I moved at a high rate of speed. All the things I did were utterly disparate. There were real highs and some real lows. Roller-coaster stomach drops and jittery fingers are just the way I like life, it turns out.

I downshifted for the last event of the day where I met Kristin van Ogtrop, the editor of *Real Simple* magazine and author of the book, *Just Let Me Lie Down: Necessary Terms for the Half-Insane Working Mom*. I introduced myself and told her what I'm sure most everyone does, something like, "I love the pretty magazine…gosh, it's amazing to think about having things organized and lovely, polite and well mannered…comparatively, my house is a dump and I work crazy hours and I love my kids' pants off every day." She mentioned how her house really isn't all *Real Simple*-ized. She said it looks a lot like other peoples' houses. She said she works a lot. She's a mom, busied and pulled all sorts of ways.

Her arms looked remarkably well attached, though.

Her book is about the insanity of working while raising kids and making sense of self-diagnosed neuroses. It's not advice.

She said things like this

- I love what I do, I love my family, I live a crazy life. *Ditto.*
- There are vulnerabilities in my children that I would never write about. *Ditto.*
- There are lots of boys around me. Lots of sports stuff. *Ditto.*
- Enjoying your work and your children in life is like how we eat: a hamburger one day, a salad the next, and it all kind of balances out. *Ditto.*

But then she gave me a Mother's Day gift without even knowing it. Unwrapped and raw, clean and short.

She explained that she was an editor, commuted to New York on the weekdays, had 3 boys at home, had just written a book. She described her friends and their formula for living and raising, working, and sleeping. She echoed something I say to parents in clinic all the time: There is no "right" formula, just one that will work for you.

Then she FedExed the gift my way.

Insanity is okay. It's great to have more (or less) commitments than people feel you should. It's okay to live a nutty life and not want to let go of any of your commitments. It's okay to like it this way.

Part 2 of the gift occurred this morning. I've been giving myself a few stolen hours here and there with the boys. I unschedule the nanny when I am supposed to work. This morning I got 2 extra hours. It was sunny with rigid lines of green and blue outside. We played with trains and airplanes. Everyone ate their breakfast.

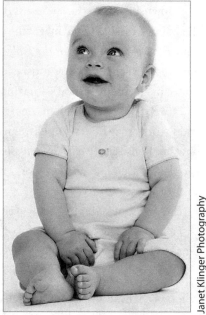

Then, for the first time ever after dropping Finn at preschool, he cried when I was leaving. Although it broke me (I cried later too), it also made me know that he feels pulled in more than one direction. He adores school, but he, too, enjoyed the morning like I did.

Everyone else keeps telling me I can't do all this. Kristin van Ogtrop and my eldest, Finn, made me know I can.

A little whiff of insanity is OK by me. Thanks for the generous gifts, Finn and Kristin. Happy Mother's Day, even if it's not the middle of May.

A baby photo of my son!

Janet Klinger Photography

WendySueSwanson MD @SeattleMamaDoc

Brutal good-bye w my 4 yo today. Sometimes he just wants mom around all day. Unsure how to avoid the pierce in my heart #worklifebalance

Getting It "Right": Birthdays in Mommyland

My quarterly crisis in work-life balance is rearing its very ugly head. See, when it's birthday season around our home, the celebrations overlap with the holiday season. I tend to feel an irrepressible need to reflect. Holidays and birthdays are momentous moments but also markers of time. Places on the calendar and spaces in my heart for subscribed reflection and perspective gathering.

It's thus at the time of year when people decorate trees and put out candles when I seem to struggle the most with my choices as a mom and a doctor, a wife and a daughter, a community member and a girl just trying to get it all "right."

I cry every year on my boys' birthdays. The tears well up out of joy (wow-wow-wow my little boys love getting older and their joy with the special day grows annually) and also out of sadness. Sadness in my ongoing strife with the question of shifting balances, purpose, goals, and daily mindfulness. Am I working too much, am I missing something, am I as present as I can be? Should I be home more? Should I contribute and write more? Should I be seeing more patients? Can I help more people than I am helping today?

I'm torn. Shred up about what is "right" (for me), and on birthdays I'm nearly emulsified. This is tough stuff. As the years tick by and the acknowledgment of mortality grows as the days seem to seep into the ether, I really want to have no regret. Sometimes, like most humans, I do.

Part of the trouble is the words of all the parents around me. They all say the exact same thing. And they have been saying it to me for more than 7 years. I know they say it to you too. The woman at the grocery store, the mentor or peer, my good friend, the doctor across the country, the parents in my clinic, my mother, the barista, the man helping me at the parking garage…they all say the exact same thing when they see my boys.

"It just goes too fast."

If you haven't heard that statement (followed by the inevitable advice), you haven't left the house with your baby/toddler/child. Or you're stuck under some big, heavy rock.

And so, as both of the boys' birthdays mixed up with Thanksgiving, Christmas, and New Year's, I become awash in the irreplaceable quandary of living life to the fullest. Valuing my boys like nothing else, I am clear on their priority in my life. I am clear about the priorities of caring for and supporting my patients. But as a friend said over the weekend, "You can't stop valuing your own life too." And part of that life includes my motherhood but also my work, my self-care, my relationships with friends, and a commitment to those around me.

And so I will sit in this space today, spinning like a top at the end of the cycle when it starts to wobble, and I'll wonder once again as the candles get blown out, am I doing it all "right"?

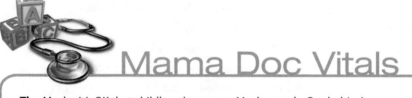

Mama Doc Vitals

Tip: Maybe it's OK that childhood moves at Mach speeds. Our babies' childhood does go fast. I think all these parents ahead of us are correct. But without the ability to stop time, it's an inevitable, inconvenient truth. Each and every day my boys get older, this really just gets better....

90

Tina Fey's Triannual Sob, the Mommy Wars, and a Truce

Tina Fey, I hear ya. As working moms, we're asked an unfair question when we are asked about "juggling it all." And I'm with you on the angst about working and parenting, except your triannual sob is my quarterly crisis.

Tina Fey, mama-again/hilarious-comedian/"ridiculously-successful-and-famous"/deserving-it-girl motherhood was once showcased in *The New York Times*. It was in the Sunday Styles section, a portion of the paper I fondly refer to as the "ladies' sports section." I can't remember who coined the nickname, but the section is defined by wedding announcements, articles about junky TV, and snapshots of random strangers carrying coffee or poodle accessories in Manhattan. But I sincerely don't mean to marginalize it. Often the section houses little storytelling gems that sit with me all week. The piece about Ms Fey got my heart pounding. There she was, one of the funniest people on the planet, saying the same things that I do. Well, kind of. Our only similarity really may be that I'm just another working mom. But it made me want to listen to her even more.

Tina, like the rest of us, is asked to defend her work, her "juggle," her parenthood differently because she's a mom. Curtis Sittenfeld writes that in Ms Fey's new book, *Bossypants,* she asserts, "'The rudest question you can ask a woman' is, 'How do you juggle it all?'" Simply put, it's archaic to think of life this way. Women are continually reminded to question their choices differently than male counterparts in the workplace even when we share parenting responsibilities. The questions alone arguably bring the working-mom struggle back to our windshields. And it ultimately perpetuates gender inequality. Why is it any different for me than it is for my husband? He works just as many hours as I do. But no one asks him about balance. Or commitment. True, this struggle really doesn't tug on him like it does on me. I believe cultural norms play a role in this.

I often talk about my quarterly working mom crisis. Well, it's not going away. Because ultimately, juggling/balancing/negotiating working and parenting is an unsolvable riddle. How to do good, feel good, work hard, parent exquisitely well, and feel comfortable with your choice, all the while enmeshed in a culture that continually asks you to question your role. Ms Fey mentions that when people ask her how she "juggles it all," she says, "Of course, I'm not supposed to admit that there is triannual torrential sobbing in my office." And then smarts, "But I have friends who stay home with their kids and they also have a triannual sob, so I think we should call it even."

A mommy wars truce, then. Perfect.

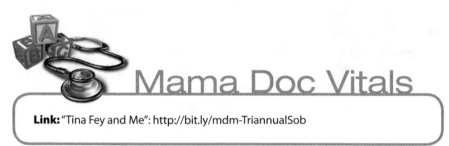

Mama Doc Vitals

Link: "Tina Fey and Me": http://bit.ly/mdm-TriannualSob

A Single Moment

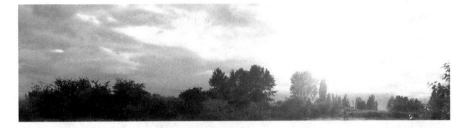

Consider this an intermission. A moment when I have no wisdom to share, no knowledge or research I'm compelled to report, and no breaking news I feel I have to detail. This is a day where those words don't come easily for me, and thus I'll give you a brief intermission. The reason? I've heard terrible news about children going missing, children who have been hurt, and children who have been killed. It's left me a bit breathless. I've found myself unable to finish 5 articles I've started writing. This past weekend I flew out to Minnesota for a 24-hour visit to support a dear friend who just lost her father. It's Wednesday now and I'm still a bit consumed by it. And more, I've been sick for the last 7 days, feeling fairly miserable. As I wring myself out and attempt to stand back up after a long week for me personally, I acknowledge this: often we lack control of all that we'd like. Everything from our own health, our family's health, the safety and vulnerability of our friends and loved ones, and even our own future.

Yet the saving grace can be that our lives can feel entirely whole in a single moment. A single moment of simplicity amid a slanted sun. The bare-bones moments away from technology and a clock—those moments surrounded by those we love. Those moments that define and then *refine* who and what we cherish most.

As the sun set last night, the boys raced between the heathers. They took small risks. They went "off road." I stood underneath a big sky, between the hill and the lake, my husband, and my 2 little boys. It was, and continues to be, a purely miraculous memory. It was just the same in the moment. The privilege to raise little boys. The joy I feel in their presence and the sincere fortune it is to watch them grow.

That is an intermission. A look into the night's golden light. A moment for you to stare at that sky too.

With that, I will heal myself, return to my patients tomorrow, and come back with much more to say.

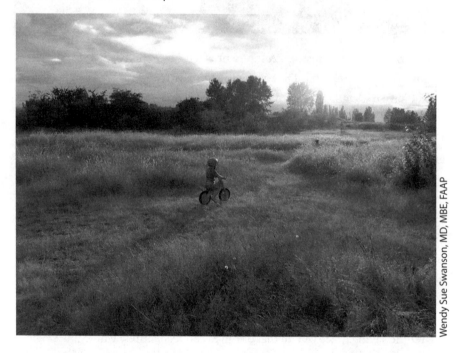

Wendy Sue Swanson, MD, MBE, FAAP

92

I Love Being a Working Mom

The social-emotional health of your child is entirely dependent on your own, at times.

I love being a working mom. The love for my work evolves, ebbs, and flows. I had one of the best days of my life in the spring of 2013, seriously ranking up there in the top 5 thus far. And unsurprisingly to me, it was a workday. However, unlike ever before, for the very first time I brought my son with me.

Every spring has "Bring Your Kid to Work Day," but really any day we do it counts. Pick an ideal time and involve your child with your work. My contention is that you'll rapidly recognize the incredible fortune it is to live this lunatic life that requires navigating the dreaded work-life–balance ordeal.

> *Pick an ideal time and involve your child with your work.*

When my 6-year-old joined me on the work trip, it was as if at once 2 huge ships met at sea. All of a sudden my little boy was welcomed into the world of making change. I felt unlike ever before that I represented more of my whole self while at work. And let me tell you, his eyes were wide open. All day.

One of the Post-it notes on my computer at home says, "Design a beautiful day." The quote stems from Marty Seligman, PhD, who's known to have founded the field of positive psychology. He devised the concept of the beautiful day activity.

Thing is, every time I've talked about designing a beautiful or meaningful day, work is a part of it. If I only had one more day to live, I'd work for a few hours in the morning. No question about it. I really do love working as a doctor. Of course, I really do love being a mom. Valuing both of these roles takes skill, and I don't always have it.

And that's the thing. I often feel like all the writing about work and balance and parenting, especially for women, causes spectators on the sideline to question a commitment toward family, children, and self for those of us also working outside of our homes. It's as if when we admit we love to nurture those outside of our family, we somehow don't value the nurturing at home as much. And it doesn't work that way in my heart.

My priorities are clearly stacked up with my children first, but one tension that I never can articulate well is the reality that I don't just work to earn money (although the paycheck is necessary); I work to get things done and to make the world more of what I know it can be.

During the spring of 2013 I gave a TED talk (TED stands for Technology, Entertainment, Design, by the way) in the Netherlands. And lucky enough for me, my 6-year-old, Finn, was in the third row. I felt more whole than I can remember feeling since returning to work after his birth. Having him at my side allowed me to feel less pull than other workdays. It's also very clear that he understands who I am in an unexpected new way.

I clearly know it's not plausible for most of us to bring our children to work most days (and it's not every day I get to do a talk in Europe!), but I encourage you, whenever you see a window, on "Bring Your Kid to Work Day" or not, bring your child to work with you. Even if just for an hour or two. Make "going to work" real, tactile, and vivid for him.

I didn't see it coming; I mean, the meaning and mindfulness of the workday with my boy. Although I had hopes that a trip to the Netherlands with Finn would be unique and cherished, I didn't understand that the long day of work was the one that would be so meaningful and so fueling. He sat through the entire day of TED talks, met dozens of colleagues, and seemed to take it all in. The talks spanned birth to death, with the morning focused on early life and the end of the day honed in on the end of life and the positive experience we can have as we age and as we die. It was heavy, but as I checked in on him throughout the day, he continued to reflect his interest and sense of calm.

It was only late at night, during pillow talk in the hotel, that I understood how profound a day with adults can be for a curious child. How essential days like this may be for curious, ready children. I was reminded not to underestimate these boys.

As he lie tucked in bed, surrounded by origami cranes he had collected during the day, he said (and I quote), "Oh, Mommy, life can be soooooooo beautiful."

"Yes, Lovey, it can," I said, my stomach flipping with surprise. And then he uttered this astonishment:

"Mommy, death can be beautiful too."

And that's when I knew, whenever possible, I had to involve my boys in my work. Share with them the luxury it is to have an education, a chance at making other people's lives better, and the fortune of a meaningful career. So nice to have the rare episode that cemented the truth—I love being a working mom.

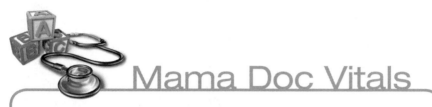

Mama Doc Vitals

Link: I mentioned this in Chapter 42, "Why the Pony Doesn't Win" (page 169) too, but here's a link on ways to complete the beautiful day activity by Marty Seligman, PhD:http://bit.ly/mdm-BeautifulDay.

93

Baby Elephants and the Working Mom

Working-mommy crises ensue regularly, yet sometimes in the most unusual form. One that I remember clearly was during my regular Thursday, a 14-hour workday away from my boys. I left the house before 7:00 am and didn't return home until nearly 9:00 pm, so consequently didn't see the boys at all that day. But that wasn't it. I was doing just fine with my day; I'd seen more than 25 patients in clinic, made some inroads on work in social media, and sincerely enjoyed the opportunities I had to help. The shift occurred after I decided to watch the first disc in the *Planet Earth* series. I popped in the DVD.

The show has nothing to do with women in the workforce. I don't think the BBC producers thought once about inspiring thoughts on work-life balance. Yet the series has everything to do with parenting, our connection to community, our space in nature, and our commitment to our children. The future of the health of our planet is dependent on our care for it now, of course. Our task in helping preserve the Earth is really about more than the quantity of plastic that ends up in landfills. It's really about how we learn to love and enjoy the woods and the wilderness, how we learn to live and travel without leaving large marks, and how our children understand what matters outside the walls of their homes. And how they come to understand decision-making.

The BBC series highlights the Earth from every contour and perspective while chronicling animals of all forms in their process of incubation (penguins = amazing), rearing, surviving, and dying.

I just kept watching the mothers. My stomach flipped at points as I watched a mother elephant help her young bull who'd walked right into a tree because he'd been blinded in a dust storm. Or the polar bear teaching her young cub to walk. These animals flanked their mothers. The babies would get tired during migration and sit down. Their mother urged them on. Even after the room was dark and I plopped into bed, I was eyes-wide-open thinking about those mothers.

No mention of fathers the entire 3 hours outside of mating rituals (I'm serious). Only the mothers, with their babes in tow, marching through the dessert, feeding after hibernation, teaching their young to walk, feed, and survive. And it struck me. Is this why this tension feels so much stronger for me? Often I'm not the one in the front of the line with my kids. I'm at clinic with other people's children. I'm writing or tweeting. I'm at a meeting. Is this struggle with balance hardwired?

It's not guilt I feel. It's far more complicated than that.

As a friend wrote today in an e-mail, "I totally go through phases of extreme despondency from missing the kids and elation at being in an exciting, fulfilling job. Don't think that a happy medium exists in real life."

Does it?

Stephen Ludwig, MD, FAAP, a cherished mentor for me during medical school, wrote and gave a lecture that was ultimately transcribed and published in *Pediatrics*. The topic was work-life balance. He talked about the struggle of raising children during his internship 38 years ago and how work-life balance is an issue for us all, but that women of childbearing age may "bear a disproportionate share" of the burden. He wants pediatricians to "strive for polygamy" and recommends that pediatricians maintain a balance and respect for 3 marriages. He discusses them in order of priority: marriage to our partners and families, marriage to our work, and marriage to ourselves. But then he adds a visual of an equally overlapping Venn diagram of these 3 unions. As pediatricians, he asserts that we need to be at the forefront of creating workplace child care (we aren't), flexible work schedules (we aren't), and vacations that span 2 weeks' time (we don't do this). We need to find ways to find silence in our lives to reflect on our biggest challenges. We need to learn to say, "No."

He ends the lecture with a Chinese philosophy.

> Happiness is someone to love,
>
> Something to do,
>
> And something to hope for.

And with that, I've found a bit more peace. But I still need to figure how to find more time to be around my little boys, in case of a dust storm.

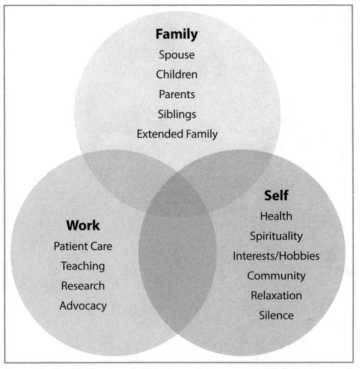

Source: Ludwig S. The Joseph W. St Geme Jr Lecture: striving for "polygamy."
Pediatrics. 2011;127(2):358–362

94

Time Magazine and the Mommy Middle Road

Have you seen that *Time* magazine cover with the 4-year-old breastfeeding while standing on a stool with the words, "Are You Mom Enough?" The day the cover came out, patients weren't talking about it in the clinic, but my e-mail inbox was piling up. I hear and feel and witness the anxiety/angst we all swim around in every day as we compare parenting styles and essentially swap (pacifier) spit about how best to do this. The monogram of this parenting era is the quest for perfection. The epic win that's constructed for us is built on prevailing over the rest. It's not about juggling it all anymore; it's about being tough enough to do it *better* than your peers. *Time* magazine wants us to contemplate if we're really "mom enough"?

> ### *I simply wish I worried less about my choices.*

Before you know it, you'll be 13 decisions down the road wondering why you worried so much about what you did. You'll care even less about what you called it. Of anything I hear over and over again from parents ahead of me on the road, it's this: "I simply wish I worried less about my choices."

It's a mom-eat-mom world right now, and the media wants us perpetually navel staring. Doubt sells magazines, page views, and books. I saw moms post opinions on Facebook about the *Time* cover only to quickly take them down as they got too controversial. We'll keep questioning ourselves and our decisions as *Time* takes a supermodel-type beauty, airbrushes her body, and paints the cover of the magazine with a provocative image for Mother's Day. This article, this cover, this timing—this is the engineering of our age. The dinosaurs once ruled the planet—now it's the voices online.

Your motherhood, your parenthood, your decisions. You know what? Of course they're mom enough…

The cover really isn't really about breastfeeding, but I'll bite. In my opinion, the decision regarding what day to stop breastfeeding is one that resides between only 2 people: a child and a mother. As an infant matures and develops coordination, independence, and new autonomy, by 1 year of age they are able to self-feed, eat and enjoy solids, and drink from a sippy or regular cup. When this occurs, the necessity for breastfeeding diminishes. Yet who am I to dictate the time to stop? As a pediatrician, it's simply not my job, as there isn't a lot of science defining the "right" deadline. And that's the exquisite gift that William Sears, MD, gave us with attachment parenting. He took the brilliance of Dr Spock and pushed a bit farther—he said we could and should attach ourselves to our babies when possible, nurture them with intimacy, and enjoy it.

Yum. I'll take a bite of that too.

Trouble is, for the working moms and the moms with multiple responsibilities, 100% attachment parenting is challenging and onerous and fills us with anxiety when we feel we fall short.

The task for all of us then, with any parenting style, is to moderate, to pick and choose the pieces and suggestions we like and leave the others behind. The real win as mothers and fathers now may be to find the middle road briskly and then live in it instead of around it, constantly questioning it.

The movement to bully moms or have moms evangelize what they do (like the aim of the *Time* cover) is far from helpful. Especially as we plan our weekend to celebrate the most extraordinary gift in our lives: the privilege of becoming a mom.

We don't have data to suggest any scarring to children who enjoy prolonged breastfeeding into their preschool years. The contrary, maybe—some breastfeeding advocates collect information about nutritional benefits for nursing past 12 months.

Point is, parenting doesn't have to feel like this. The pulse of our response (whatever yours is) to the image of a gorgeous woman nursing her near 4-year-old really isn't so much about attachment parenting or not, breastfeeding past infancy or not, swaddling or not, peas before carrots or not; the pulse to this cover and the viral mommy war and guilt that ensue is about much more. It's really about the ongoing construct that the media has created to have us believe that this tension/discourse/doubt/mommy "war" is what parenting should feel like.

Turn off the computer; throw out the books. Enjoy the choices you've made and move on. Bear witness to the ultimate luxury of life: the gift of your child.

Online Resources for Parents

In no way is this list comprehensive. I've clearly had to leave some very notable voices out (please accept my apologies)! But if you follow these folks, they will surely lead you the right ways. And when fresh, incredible, unexpected voices arrive on the scene that can improve your life, these people will help remind us they are here.

Blogs and Bloggers I Like

www.boston.com/lifestyle/health/mdmama
http://kckidsdoc.com
www.huffingtonpost.com/lisa-belkin
www.weightymatters.ca
http://susannahfox.com
http://joycelee.tumblr.com
www.33charts.com
http://sethmnookin.com/
http://parenting.blogs.nytimes.com
http://mytwohats.com
www.confessionsofadrmom.com
www.emilywillinghamphd.com
www.sethgodin.com
www.seattlemamadoc.com (That's me!)

Twitter

Parenting Voices
@LizSzabo
@phdinparenting
@micheleborba
@LesbianDad
@lisabelkin
@dooce
@RichLouv
@TheMamaFesto
@scienceofmom
@Voices4Vaccines
@AdamsLisa
@mindthecompany
@parentsmagazine
@SolidFooting

Pediatrician-Moms to Follow
@drClaire
@DoctorNatasha
@DrKimMD
@DrMommyCalls
@baby411
@LivingWellDoc
@Melissa_DrMom
@drlaurajana
@DrAlannaLevine
@MDPartner
@DrIvorHorn
@KateLandMD
@MomDocKathleen
@hkroman
@safetymd (pediatric emergency medicine, prevention)
@Kind4Kids
@TheKidsDoctor
@KPkiddoc

@joyclee (pediatric endocrinology, technology)
@drsilva_kids
@drmlb (pediatric surgeon)
@mommy_call

Pediatrician and Family-Doc Dads to Follow
@parikhmd
@DrCanapari (pediatric sleep medicine)
@rychoiMD
@drflanders
@drpauldempsey
@ChrisCarrollMD
@davhill
@aaronecarroll (health economics, pediatrics)
@Doctor_V (pediatric gastroenterology, technology)
@KidsDrDave
@PMillerMD
@ChrisJohnsonMD (critical care pediatrics, general pediatrics)
@DrGreene
@YoniFreedhoff (obesity, nutrition)
@DrStephenPont (obesity, general pediatrics)
@CountryKidsDoc

Broadcasting Good Health Information and Opinion
@kevinmd
@sethmnookin
@HonestToddler (humor)
@drcindyhaines
@garyschwitzer
@Dermdoc
@cslnyt
@DrRichardBesser
@debkotz2
@healthychildren

For Expecting Mothers and Fathers
@CatchTheBaby

@DrJenGunter

On Health and Technology
@EricTopol

@SusannahFox

@rzeiger

@ahier

Facebook

Health Information
SeattleMamaDoc

    www.facebook.com/SeattleMamaDoc

Voices For Vaccines

    www.facebook.com/VoicesForVaccines

PKIDs (Parents of Kids with Infectious Diseases)

    www.facebook.com/PKIDsOnline

The Car Seat Lady

    www.facebook.com/TheCarSeatLady

Common Sense Media

    www.facebook.com/commonsensemedia

Healthy Children

    www.facebook.com/healthychildren

Standout Pediatrician Practice Pages I Like
KC Kids Doc

    www.facebook.com/Pediatric.Associates.Kansas.City

Kids Plus Pediatrics

    www.facebook.com/KidsPlusPediatrics

Dr. Kim's Kids (Winnsboro Pediatrics)

    www.facebook.com/pages/Dr-Kims-Kids-Winnsboro-Pediatrics/
    144803248887013

Other Web Sites

General Parenting Information
www.HealthyChildren.org
www.nlm.nih.gov/medlineplus/childrenshealth.html
http://well.blogs.nytimes.com/category/family-2/18-and-under

Food Allergies
www.foodallergy.org

Television, Video Games, Ratings, and Advice on Media
www.commonsensemedia.org

Information for Children With Gastrointestinal Diseases
www.gikids.org

Information for Parents and Children With Infectious Diseases
www.pkids.org

Vaccines
www.chop.edu/service/vaccine-education-center
www.nnii.org
www.cdc.gov/vaccines/hcp/vis
www.immunize.org

Concussions
http://Cdcheadsup.org

Sports and Screening for Sudden Cardiac Death
www.nickoftimefoundation.org
www.parentheartwatch.org

Index